EXPERIENTIAL LEARNING IN ACTION

For John Heron and Peter Jarvis
Two different sorts of humanistic educators

Experiential Learning in Action

PHILIP BURNARD
University of Wales College of Medicine

Avebury

Aldershot · Brookfield USA · Hong Kong · Singapore · Sydney

Published by
Avebury
Academic Publishing Group
Gower House
Croft Road
Aldershot
Hants GU11 3HR
England

Gower Publishing Company
Old Post Road
Brookfield
Vermont 05036
USA

A CIP catalogue record for this book is available from
the British Library and the US Library of Congress.

ISBN 1 85628 261 9

Printed and Bound in Great Britain by
Athenaeum Press Ltd., Newcastle upon Tyne.

Contents

Acknowledgements

Thanks go to a number of people whose help and support was appreciated during the research described here and during the writing process. First and particularly, to Professor Jillian Macquire, for her patient help, advice, encouragement and enthusiasm. Thank you.

Second, thanks to Professor Peggy Anne Field, University of Alberta, Edmonton, for her advice on questionnaire design and research methodology and for her helpful comments.

Particular thanks go to my colleague Paul Morrison for his friendship, advice and support at all times and to Sandy Kirkman for her friendship and all her help. Finally, particular thanks, as ever, to my wife Sally and to my children, Aaron and Rebecca who put up with a great deal, who complained only occasionally and who were always encouraging. Especial thanks to Aaron, who has patiently taught me about computing.

About the author

Philip Burnard is Director of Postgraduate Nursing Studies at the University of Wales College of Medicine, Cardiff, Wales, UK and Honourary Lecturer in Nursing at the Hogeschool Midden Nederland, Utrecht, Netherlands. He has a Master of Science degree in educational studies from the University of Surrey and a PhD in experiential learning from the University of Wales. He is also a qualified general and mental health nurse. He has published 11 textbooks on interpersonal skills, counselling, education, ethics and research and published numerous papers on these topics. Dr Burnard's research interests include teaching and learning styles, nurses' training needs in the field of AIDS counselling and attitudes towards counselling styles. He is married with two children and lives in Caerphilly, South Wales.

Introduction

If you want to know what someone is about, ask them -
they might just tell you.
George Kelly

We all learn from experience : at least some of the time. The term
"experiential learning" has been widely used in nursing education but
not always clearly defined. The aim of this study was to attempt to
clarify the concept of experiential learning as it relates to education.
The study described in this book uses nursing education as a case
study. The findings of the study have relevance for all types of
education : from secondary to higher for experiential learning methods
are used throughout the educational system in various forms.

Experiential learning methods have been recommended for use
in helping nurses to develop interpersonal skills in nursing (Kagan 1985,
Kagan, Kay and Evans, 1985, Raichura 1987) . One of the most explicit
recommendations for their use was in the 1982 syllabus of training for
psychiatric nursing students (ENB 1982). This was an unusual step for,
as Kelly (1977) noted, syllabi do not usually prescribe teaching and
learning methods but normally only indicate the content of courses.
Prior to and following the publication of the syllabus, there were a
number of publications relating to the use of experiential learning

1

methods in psychiatric nurse education (Dietrich 1978, Bailey 1983, Burnard 1983, Dowd 1983).

Since those early papers, a number of other papers appeared in the literature on the use of experiential learning as an approach to teaching nursing (Miles 1987,Sankar 1987, Raichura 1987). The approach was also recommended in a learning package published by the English National Board for Nursing, Midwifery and Health Visiting, Managing Change in Nurse Education (ENB 1987). Given the variety of writing that was available on the use of experiential learning in psychiatric and general nursing it was decided to explore the concept in both disciplines.

In exploring the field both theoretically and practically, it became clear that experiential learning was understood and used in a variety of ways. Sometimes it appeared to be a discrete learning method (Kolb 1984) and at other times it seemed to be more of a series of learning techniques that had developed out of the school of humanistic psychology (Shaffer 1978, Rowan 1988). Some "ground clearing" work was planned. It was reasoned that if tutors themselves experienced a certain confusion of what was to be understood by the term "experiential learning", then it was possible that the students being taught by those tutors might experience some confusion. Thus the present study was devised.

The study was a descriptive one which combined qualitative and quantitative methods to identify a range of perceptions of two groups of people : nurse tutors and nursing students. A series of semi-structured interviews were used to explore perceptions and transcripts of these interviews were analysed using content analysis and a modified "grounded theory" approach (Glaser and Strauss 1967, Strauss 1986).

Out of these findings, a questionnaire was developed and a larger group of nurse tutors and student nurses was surveyed to examine the degree to which a larger sample endorsed or did not endorse the initial findings. From these findings, it was possible to develop theoretical and practical models for nurse education.

The book is laid out as follows. Chapter one offers a review of the literature regarding experiential learning, experiential learning methods and experiential learning in nurse education. Chapter two identifies the research design and the methodology. Chapter three describes the qualitative study of tutors' and students' perceptions of experiential learning. Chapters four and five offer the findings from the initial analysis of the tutors' and students' interviews. Chapters six

2

and seven offer the findings from the secondary analyses. Chapter eight describes the survey carried out with a larger sample and chapter nine identifies the findings from that survey. Chapter ten compares and contrasts the findings from the interviews and from the questionnaire. Chapter eleven reviews the study, offers evaluative comment and identifies some limitations. The final chapter offers a discussion of the findings with recommendations for practice and future research.

The term "tutor" is widely used to describe those actively involved in teaching student nurses. At times, other descriptors are used, both in the literature and by the tutors themselves. Whilst the term "tutor" is used most frequently throughout this book, occasionally the terms "educator", "facilitator" or "lecturer" are used when appropriate. The terms "he" and "his" are used in the discussion of the interview data so that respondents cannot be identified.

Background to the Study

This section is the "biography of the study". It identifies the researcher's disposition towards experiential learning at the start of the study. Research does not occur in a vacuum and is not carried out by objective, detached workers who are ahistorical. As Weiss and Kempler (1986) indicate, in all psychological and educational research, the researcher's personal intent always has a bearing on the research design and on the outcome. The aim of this section is to declare the researcher's interest in the topic and to show how I attempted to overcome biases.

I became a tutor, in psychiatric nursing, at the end of the 1970's as the new psychiatric nursing syllabus was being developed. When the 1982 syllabus was issued in draft and finally complete form, various workshops in experiential learning methods were offered at the Human Potential Research Project, University of Surrey, Guildford. Through such workshops, I developed a range of facilitation skills and a critical theoretical base within the field of experiential learning. This base was elaborated through a Master of Science in Education degree in the Department of Education, University of Surrey. Whilst this was a broad based, taught master's degree in various aspects of the education of adults, I was able to concentrate on studying various humanistic approaches to learning and also on the theory and practice of experiential learning.

This theoretical and practical training and education was put into practice in my work as a nurse tutor. A variety of papers on practical and theoretical aspects of experiential learning in the nursing and educational journals followed (e.g.Burnard 1983, 1984, 1986, 1987a, 1988a, 1988b 1989a) and two books on the topic (Burnard 1985, 1989c).

A change of job to Lecturer in Nursing at the University of Wales College of Medicine, Cardiff, further work on the topic and the opportunity to explore the use of experiential learning methods in Canada and the USA via a Florence Nightingale scholarship (Burnard 1987b), led to certain questions. Why was there so little research into the use of experiential learning in nursing? Did it "work"? Finally, and most pertinent to the present study : what **was** experiential learning? It seemed that this question needed to be addressed before work could be done on the efficiency or otherwise of experiential learning.

In the years leading up to and during this study, experiential learning tended to generate "converts" : nurse tutors who tended to identify closely with the field of experiential learning (the word "converts" is used advisedly and this is returned to in the final chapter). They tended to emphasis certain values : individuality, the development of self, the need for negotiation in the curriculum, the primacy of students' personal experience and so forth. In a way, they have their parallel in the world of research. They are in some ways similar to that group of researchers who stress the importance of **qualitative** methods over and against quantitative methods. Just as the advocates of qualitative research sometimes seem to suggest that qualitative methods are "right" and preferable to quantitative methods (Leininger 1985 is an example of one such nurse researcher), so some advocates of experiential learning tend to suggest that the experiential approach is the most appropriate way of teaching and learning. Those people tend to be scathing of what they see as the more traditional and restrictive educational practices (an example of this sort of "evangelism" can be found in Rowan 1988).

Whilst acknowledging the apparent practical value of certain experiential learning methods in teaching interpersonal skills, I was less certain about the validity of the "two camps" debate about whether or not experiential learning was a "better" or more appropriate approach to nurse education. I am not claiming that I occupy a detached and objective position vis a vis this project, nor am I blind to the lack of empirical evidence to support the use of the

4

experiential learning approach. I felt that there was considerable lack of uniformity about how experiential learning was to be defined. It was too early to try to identify whether or not experiential learning was an "effective" method of learning. Instead, some clarifying work needed to be done in order to try to find out how both tutors and students perceived experiential learning. This book attempts to clarify the field a little by laying out and analysing the perceptions of both those who claim to use an experiential learning approach and experiential learning methods and those who are subject to them.

Certain considerations and assumptions were made during the development and writing of this book. First, an attempt was made to rigorously analyse the data developed out of interviews and questionnaires. Second, a book is a form of communication with other people and should be **readable**. This thought developed from C. Wright Mill's remark that, "To overcome the academic **prose** you have first to overcome the academic pose" (Wright Mills : 1959 . 66). In reviewing some of the literature on writing (Turk and Kirkman 1989, Palmer and Pope 1984, Brande 1981, Turabian 1987), it became evident that many academics confuse a heavy and turgid writing style with academic excellence. I have tried to develop a straightforward and readable style that combines both the description of the respondent's thoughts and perceptions with the necessary development of theory out of those perceptions.

1 Experiential learning: Definitions, descriptions and theories

This chapter reviews some of the literature on experiential learning and, given the accent on the use of experiential learning, refers to the literature on experiential learning in nursing.

Introduction

How do people learn to become nurses? One approach is through the use of our own experience via experiential learning methods. In this chapter experiential learning is explored through the literature. The discussion of the relevant literature is also developed throughout the analysis of the data, in chapters 5 - 7 and in the final chapters in which the findings are discussed.

The Development of the Concept of Experiential Learning

People have always learned from experience. However, the idea of experiential learning as an educational concept is a relatively recent one. The first part of this chapter traces the historical roots of experiential learning.

Developing the work of American pragmatic philosopher, John Dewey (1916, 1938), Keeton and Associates (1976) described experiential learning as including learning through the process of living and included work experience, skills developed through hobbies and interests and non-formal educational activities. This approach was reflected in the Further Education Unit project report "Curriculum Opportunity" which asserted that experiential learning referred to the knowledge and skills acquired through life and work experience and study (F.E.U. 1983).

Pfeiffer and Goodstein (1982) took a different approach by describing an "experiential learning cycle" which spelt out the process of experiential learning (Figure 1.1) This cycle not only suggested the format for organising experiential learning but also made tacit reference to the way
in which people learn through experience.

1. Experiencing
2. Publishing (Sharing reactions and experiences)
3. Processing (Discussion
of patterns and dynamics)
4. Generalising (Inferring
principles about the "real world")
5. Applying (Planning more effective behaviour)

Figure 1.1 Experiential Learning Cycle (After Pfeiffer and Goodstein 1982)

Kolb (1984) was more explicit about this learning process in his "experiential learning model" (Figure 1.2). In this model, concrete experience was the starting point for a reflective process that echoed Paulo Freire's (1972) concept of "praxis". Praxis, for Freire was the combination of reflection-and-action-in-the-world : a transforming process that is one of man's distinguishing features and one that enables him to change his view of the world and ultimately, to change the world itself.

1. Concrete Experience
2. Observations
3. Formation of abstract concepts and generalisations
4. Testing implications of and reflections on concepts in new situations.

Figure 1.2: Experiential Learning Cycle (After Kolb 1984)

Kolb's model is not dissimilar to the Action Learning cycle described by Garrett (1983) and illustrated in Figure 1.3. Action Learning was an approach to learning in the field of organisational and business psychology by Revans (Revans 1978, 1982) and designed to help to generate solutions to real-life problems. It was defined by Pedlar (1983) as follows :

> Action Learning is a development process in which individuals learn through attempting organisational change by tackling hitherto intractable problems in the company of four or five others. (Pedlar 1983 :2).
> As in experiential learning, the emphasis in Action Learning is on the concrete experience of the individuals taking part in the learning activity.

Like experiential learning, Action Learning depended on the process of reflection.

1. Observation
2. Reflection
3. Hypothesis
4. Reflection
5. Action

Figure 1.3: The Action Learning Cycle (after Garratt 1983)

Reflectivity in the learning process was developed in the educational literature (Boud, Keogh and Walker 1985, Walker, 1985, Main 1985). Grundy (1982) described how reflectivity takes place in various aspects of the experiential learning cycle. Each person, interacting with others in a learning group brings their informed practical judgement to bear on ideas relevant to the event. This episode of researching and evaluating ideas is an example of reflection in Grundy's view. A further phase of reflection may occur to re-examine more basic assumptions and deeper insights may develop. These new insights may then be applied to the original event or to similar relevant events and thus to more reflective activity. This form of reflectivity has much in common with John Dewey's definition of **reflective thought** :

> Active, persistent and careful consideration of any belief or supposed form of knowledge in the light of the grounds that support it and further conclusions to which it leads... it includes a conscious and voluntary effort to establish belief upon a firm basis of evidence and rationality. (Dewey 1933 : 9).

Indeed, Dewey might almost have been describing a major part of Kolb's experiential learning cycle. Many of the ideas about experiential learning can be traced back to Dewey's work. This is hardly suprising given that much of the original work on experiential learning is American and given that Dewey had much to do with the foundations of the American educational system (Jarvis 1984).

Powell (1985) developed the reflective diary or journal as a means of enabling students to both reflect on their learning processes and as a way of recording new learning. In a nursing context, the use of journals has been described as an assessment and evaluation tool for nursing students (Burnard 1988c).

Steinaker and Bell (1979) offered an experiential taxonomy. Five levels were described by the taxonomy (Figure 1.4). At the first level, the learner becomes conscious of an experience. At the participation level, that learner has to decide whether or not to take part in that experience. At the third level, the student becomes immersed in the experience both intellectually and emotionally. At level four, the student begins to absorb the learning that takes place and makes it his or her own. Finally, the learner, having internalised the learning from experience, shares it with others. This taxonomy of stages in the learning process has much in common with Kolb's experiential learning cycle (Kolb, 1984), described in this chapter and it has been applied to teaching and learning in nursing by Kenworthy and Nicklin (1989). They suggested that the taxonomy can be used as the basis of curriculum planning in nursing courses.

1. Exposure level,

2. Participation level,

3. Identification level,

4. Internalisation level

5. Dissemination level.

Figure 1.4 Experiential Taxonomy (Steinaker and Bell 1979)

Malcolm Knowles, the American adult educator (Knowles, 1980) took a different approach to the definition of experiential learning. He described the activities following activities as "participatory experiential techniques' :

> Group discussion, cases, critical incidents, simulations, role-play, skills practice exercises, field projects, action projects, laboratory methods, consultative supervision (coaching), demonstrations, seminars, work conferences, counselling, group therapy and community development. (Knowles 1980 : 50)

His list seems so all-inclusive that he seems to have been saying that experiential learning techniques excluded only the lecture method or private, individual study and that experiential learning was synonymous with participant and discovery learning.

Boydel (1976) described experiential learning in the following way :

> Experiential learning in general terms is synonymous with meaningful discovery learning. This is learning which involves the learner sorting things out for himself by restructuring his perceptions of what is happening. (Boydell 1976 : 19)

Summarising the position adopted by those writers who devised their definitions of experiential learning from the work of Dewey, would involve noting first the accent on a cycle of events starting with concrete experience. Kolb's and Pfeiffer and Goodstein's cycles were anticipated by Dewey himself:

Thinking includes all of these steps, the sense of a problem, the observation of conditions, the formation and rational elaboration of a suggested conclusion and the active experimental testing. (Dewey 1916 : 151).

The idea of learning from experience being a cycle involving action and reflection was a theme frequently echoed amongst modern writers (see, for example : Kelly 1977, Hampden Turner 1966). Kolb's notion of transformation of experience and meaning can also be traced back to Dewey. He wrote that :

In a certain sense every experience should do something to prepare a person for later experiences of a deeper and more expansive quality. That is the very meaning of growth, continuity, reconstruction of experience. (Dewey 1938 : 47)

This was the influence on experiential learning from the Dewey perspective. The accent was on the primacy of personal experience and on reflection as the tool for changing knowledge and meaning.

Boud and Pascoe (1978) summed up what they considered to be the most important characteristics of experiential education thus:

1. The involvement of each individual student in his or her own learning (learning activities need to engage the full attention of a student),

2. The correspondence of the learning activity to the world outside the classroom of the educational institution (the emphasis being on the quality of the experience, not its location),

3. Learner control over the learning experience (learners themselves need to have control over the experience in which they are engaged so that they can integrate it with their own mode of operation in the world and can experience the results of their own decisions). (Boud and Pascoe 1978 : 36)

Boud and Pascoes' list seems to sum up the Dewey approach to learning through experience and through responsibility in the learning process.

It was Carl Rogers who offered the clearest definition of what experiential or "significant" learning might be. He identified these elements of experiential learning :

1. It has the quality of personal involvement,
2. It is self-initiated,
3. It is pervasive,
4. It is evaluated by the learner [rather than by educators]
5. Its essence is meaning. (Rogers 1972 : 276).

Whilst the final element ("its essence is meaning") is rather unclear, Rogers' view of experiential learning was a view of "personalised" learning, which he contrasted with "cognitive learning" or the learning of facts and figures that are imposed by educators. Experiential learning, for Rogers, was learning that was self-initiated and in which the learner's interest and motivation was high. He went on to identify "assumptions relevant to experiential learning" :

1. Human beings have a natural potentiality for learning,
2. Significant learning takes place when the subject matter is perceived by the student as having relevance for his own purposes,
3. Much significant learning is acquired through doing,
4. Learning is facilitated when the student participates responsibly in the learning process,
5. Self-initiated learning, involving the whole person of the learner - feelings as well as intellect - is the most pervasive and lasting,
6. Creativity in learning is best facilitated when self-criticism and self-evaluation are primary, and evaluation by others is of secondary importance,
7. The most socially useful learning in the modern world is the learning of the process of learning, a continuing openness to experience, an incorporation into oneself of the process of change. (Rogers 1972 : 278 - 279).

It is important to note that Rogers was offering a set of **value statements** about learning as well as a list of what he saw as significant in experiential learning. Rogers' statements were based only on his experience as an educator and not on empirical evidence.

12

Carl Rogers was an important figure in the field of humanistic psychology, which is the next domain under consideration, here.

Humanistic Psychology

Humanistic psychology was an important influence on the development of experiential learning. It developed in the 1940's, 50's and 60's as a reaction to the "mechanism" of behavioural psychology and the determinism of psychodynamic psychology. Humanistic psychologists argued that people were free to choose their own lives and thus were "authors" of their own existence. This philosophical perspective drew heavily on the existentialism of Sartre (1955), Heidegger (1927) and others.

Humanistic psychology's main leaders, particularly in the 1960's (which offered exactly the right climate in which humanistic psychology could flourish) were Carl Rogers (1967, 1972, 1952) and Abraham Maslow (1972) [who is said to have named humanistic psychology (Grossman 1985)]. Rogers is particularly well known for his client-centred counselling and for his student-centred learning methods (Rogers 1983). In the 1960's he also developed the encounter group approach to developing self awareness. As we have noted, many of the experiential learning methods described here developed out of the school of humanistic psychology, which, rather like Deweyian educational practices, emphasised the uniqueness of human experience and human interpretation of the world. Rogers had been considerably influenced by Dewey as he had been taught at university by a student of Dewey's, William Kilpatrick (Kirschenbaum 1979).

The "Articles of Association" formulated by the American Association of Humanistic Psychology at its inception in 1962 described the field in this way :

> Humanistic psychology is primarily an orientation towards the whole of psychology rather than a distinct area or school. It stands for the respect and the worth of persons, respect of differences or approach, open-mindedness as to acceptable methods, and interest in exploration of new aspects of human behaviour. As a "third" force in contemporary psychology, it is concerned with **topics that have little place in existing theories and systems**   [emphasis added] : love,

13

creativity, self, growth, organism, basic need-gratification, higher values, being, becoming, play, humour, affection, naturalness, warmth, ego-transcendence, objectivity, autonomy, responsibility, meaning, fair play, transcendental experience, peak experience, courage **and related concepts** [emphasis added]. (A.A.H.P. 1962 : 2)

These were extravagant claims. Many of the "topics that have had little place in existing theories and systems" had received the attention of psychologists prior to the formation of the association (presumably, too, concepts such as "being", "objectivity" and "autonomy" had been discussed by philosophers for centuries). By way of example, in psychology, Adler (1927), Horney (1937) and Fromm (1957) had discussed love from the point of view of psychodynamic theory. Creativity had been fairly thoroughly explored by other psychologists (Getzels and Jackson 1962, Anderson 1959). Jung had used the term "self-actualisation" prior to its use in humanistic psychology (Jung 1931) and William James had examined "peak experiences" and transcendental states in a thorough work at the turn of the century (James 1902). The tone of the much of the writing in humanistic psychology is American. Yalom, writing in the late 70's, notes that :

An importation and an Americanization of existential thought and therapeutic procedure has occurred. The frame is European but the accent is unmistakably New World-ish. The Europeans focus is on the tragic dimensions of existence, on limits on facing and taking into oneself the anxiety or uncertainty and non-being. The humanistic psychologists speak less of limits and contingency than of development of potential, less of acceptance than of awareness, less of anxiety than of peak experience... (Yalom 1977 : 60-61).

Other critics were rather more direct when discussing humanistic psychology's approach. Clare described the humanistic psychology movement as part of the "me generation" culture (Clare 1981). Masson (1990) suggested that Carl Rogers was responsible for producing therapists who were "the bland showing the not-so-bland how to be bland" and accused Rogers of being politically naive.

14

It has been argued that there are at least **two** types of humanistic psychology (Rowan 1989, Mahrer 1989). One is the sort that has a particularly positive view of human beings. People are viewed as having a tendency to "grow" and develop. At its most extreme, this approach argues that people are essentially "good" : an idea that dates back at least to Rousseau. It is an idea that has tended to be a reaction against the Protestant and Freudian idea of people as essentially "evil" or bad (Murphy and Kovach 1972). This "positive" view of humanistic psychology is typified by writers such as Carl Rogers (1952, 1967) and Abraham Maslow (1972).

The second type of humanistic psychology draws more particularly from existentialism and sees people as neither good nor bad. People, in this version, are completely free. That freedom does not necessarily lead them towards goodness or badness. Essentially, people are "neutral". Representative writers of this approach include Rollo May (1989) and Erich Fromm (1957, 1979).

Both types of humanistic psychology acknowledge that people are complex and ever changing. No one theory of how people "work" would necessarily explain this person in this situation. Humanistic psychology places great importance on how the individual interprets her world and does not seek to develop a "grand theory" of how human beings think, feel and act. Thus it differs from behaviourism and psychoanalysis which both offer overall explanatory theories of the person.

In a study attempting to identify the core features of a humanistic approach to education, Shapiro (1985) identified fifteen "major operating value principles" from "40 representative and well-known humanistic educators" (unspecified). The fifteen include many of the concepts so far discussed in relation to both experiential learning in general and humanistic psychology and its relation to education in particular. Shapiro's value principles were :

   1. Process orientation,
   2. Self-determination,
   3. Connectedness,
   4. Relevancy,
   5. Integration,
   6. Awareness of context,
   7. Affective,
   8. Innovation,
   9. Democratic participation,
 10. Personal growth orientation,

11. People-oriented,
12. Individualism,
13. Reality claims,
14. Evaluation,
15. Variety-creativity.
(Shapiro 1985 : 99)

The problems with such a listing are various. First, many of the values identified here may not be exclusive to a humanistic approach to education. Most tutors would, for example, be concerned with evaluation and relevancy. Some of the values are far from clear. It would be possible to question, for example, what was meant by the term "reality claims". On the other hand, the list illustrates particular aspects of the humanistic approach to education. First, its emphasis on self and on individualism. Second, its grounding in the language of the 1960's ("connectedness"; "people-oriented"). This issue is addressed, again, in the final chapter of this book.

Butterworth (1984) proposed a set of principles that should, in his view, form a structure for a humanistic approach to nurse training. The humanistic course, should, according to Butterworth, be based on the following principles :

● it should be person-centred rather than patient-centred,
● it should facilitate personal growth through humanistic methods,
● it should examine characteristics of a helping relationship,
● learning should be a shared experience. (Butterworth 1984 : 65 - 66)

Here we see the incorporation of many of the "themes" from humanistic psychology being considered for application in the training of nurses. Butterworth went on to suggest that teaching methods in his proposed model for teaching psychiatric nurses should include ; formal teaching, seminars, discussions, experiential learning, group method experiences and "case work and supervision". Butterworth appears to have combined the experiential learning approach with more traditional teaching techniques.

The influence of humanistic psychology was clearly evident in the 1982 RMN syllabus of training for psychiatric nursing students. The syllabus contained reference to such concepts as :"the humanistic approach to psychiatric nursing practice" and "the use of self as a therapeutic agent", which were not found in previous syllabi. Also, the

16

syllabus was unequivocal in its support for the use of experiential learning methods such as the ones described in this chapter and by spondents later in the study :

> The use of experiential techniques including structured exercises, games and role play, which involve the student and his whole experience are to be recommended...

> Theoretical inputs like lectures from staff, students and outside specialists can be followed by experiential workshops related to the topic concerned. (ENB 1982 p1).

The humanistic influence can be traced to some of the members of the working party which devised the new syllabus. One member was a director of the Human Potential Research Project at the University of Surrey, one of the first "growth centres" established in the UK (Rowan 1988). Other members had attended courses of training in experiential learning methods at that department. The department had, over the years, added a significant amount to the literature on humanistic psychology in the UK. (see, for example, Heron 1975, 1977a, 1977b, 1978, Kilty 1983, Bond and Kilty 1983). This humanistic influence also became evident in the nursing literature on experiential learning that emerged around the time of, or following, the publication of the 1982 syllabus (Dietrich 1978, Kilty 1983, Burnard 1985). Arguably, the curriculum working party members were also reflecting a tendency in psychiatric nursing towards the humanistic approach to care.

In this way, we begin to develop a sense of experiential learning's heritage : American, (although drawing, also, from European philosophical traditions), with a heavy emphasis on personal experience, personal development and being influenced by the school of humanistic psychology.

The "Four Villages" Approach to Experiential Learning

Widening the debate about experiential learning even further, Weil and McGill (1989) argued that it was useful to consider the theory and practice of experiential learning by reference to a metaphor of four villages. They suggested that experiential learning theorists appeared to hold four distinct points of view (or inhabit four different villages). They went on to suggest that the people in each of those four villages tended to be unaware of the existence of the other three. They quote (from an unknown source) as follows:

> A person who knows only his own village will not understand it; only by seeing what is familiar in the light of what is the norm elsewhere will we be enabled to think afresh about what we know too well. (Weil and McGill 1989 : 4)

Weil and Mcgill suggest that we would do well not to become too narrow minded about what experiential learning is and what it is not. The four "villages" that they describe are as follows:

Village one

The assessment and accreditation of "prior" experiential learning. Essentially, the people in this village view experiential learning as learning from life experience and learning that can be "totted up" to enable adults to gain exemption from certain degree and diploma courses. In the U.K. for example, nurses who have not got "first" degrees can sometimes gain entrance to master's degree courses by virtue of their previous personal and professional experience.

Village two

Experiential learning and change in higher and continuing eduction. In this village, experiential learning is often tied closely to adult learning theory and the notion of developing learner-centred approaches to teaching and learning.

Village three

Experiential learning and social change. In this village, experiential learning is a radical process concerned with helping people to change the circumstances in which they find themselves. In this sense, it is more akin to Freire's (1972) "problem-posing" approach to education, described elsewhere in this chapter and has a "political" aspect to it.

Village four

Personal growth and development. Here, the emphasis is on the individual's learning processes and the people of this village are often aligned with the humanistic school of psychology. It is arguable that it is this "village" that has most strongly influenced the development of experiential learning in nurse education.

Weil and McGill's argument, then, is that we can learn much from **all** approaches to experiential learning - from the political aspect of it, from the adult learning approach, as well as from the personal growth and development aspect.

Experiential Learning as the Development of Experiential Knowledge

Another approach to experiential learning comes through discussion of types of knowledge. Three types of knowledge that go to make up an individual have been described by Heron (1981), a British philosopher whose work may be clearly placed within the context of humanistic psychology (see, for example, Heron 1973, 1977a, 1977b, 1986). Those types of knowledge are : propositional, practical and experiential and have been developed, in a nursing context, by the researcher (Burnard 1987a). Whilst each of the types of knowledge that Heron describes is different, each is interrelated with the other. Thus, whilst propositional knowledge may be considered as qualitatively different to, say, practical knowledge, it is possible to use propositional knowledge in the application of practical knowledge.

Propositional knowledge

Propositional knowledge is that which is contained in theories or models. It may be described as "textbook" knowledge and is synonymous with Ryle's (1949) concept of "knowing that", which is further developed in an educational context by Pring (1976). Thus a person may build up a considerable bank of facts, theories or ideas about a subject, person or thing, without necessarily having any direct experience of that subject, person or thing. A person, may, for example develop a considerable propositional knowledge about, say, midwifery, without ever necessarily having been anywhere near a

19

woman who is having a baby. Presumably it would be more useful to combine that knowledge with some practical experience, but this does not necessarily have to be the case. This, then, is the domain of propositional knowledge. Obviously it is possible to have propositional knowledge about a great number of subject areas ranging from mathematics to literature or from counselling to social work. Any information contained in books must necessarily be of the propositional sort.

Practical knowledge

Practical knowledge is knowledge that is developed through the acquisition of skills. Driving a car or giving an injection demonstrates practical knowledge. So does the use of counselling skills which involve the use of specific verbal and non-verbal behaviours and intentional use of counselling interventions. Practical knowledge is synonymous with Ryle's (1949) concept of "knowing how" which was further developed, in an educational context by Pring (1976). Usually more than mere "knack", practical knowledge is the substance of a smooth performance of a practical or interpersonal skill. Traditionally, most educational programmes in schools and colleges have concerned themselves primarily with both propositional and practical knowledge and particularly the former (Lawton 1973). Such an emphasis on the cognitive development of the person may be traced back to the classical educational system proposed by Plato : a tradition continued by a number of modern educational philosophers (Peters 1972, Perry 1972). Practical knowledge, although respected, is usually seen as slightly less important than the propositional sort. This "lop-sided" approach to education may best be illustrated in the twentieth century by reference to the Butler Education Act (HMSO 1944) which suggested that "more able" schoolchildren should receive a "grammar" (i.e. "cognitive" or academic) education, whereas less able children should receive a "secondary modern" (i.e. practical) education. Butler also recommended the development of a range of "technical" schools as an in-between placement for children falling between the secondary modern schools on the one hand and the grammar schools on the other. In practice, few technical schools were built or developed.

Experiential knowledge

The domain of experiential knowledge is knowledge gained through direct encounter with a subject, person or thing and which has an effect on self-concept. It is the subjective and affective nature of that encounter that contributes to this sort of knowledge. Experiential knowledge is knowledge through relationship. Such knowledge is synonymous with Roger's (1983) description of experiential learning and similar to Polanyi's concept of "personal" knowledge and "tacit" knowledge (Polanyi 1958). Polanyi suggests that we "know more than we can say". If we reflect for a moment we may discover that most of the things that are really important to us belong in this domain. If for example we consider our personal relationships with other people, we discover that what we like or love about them cannot be reduced to a series of propositional statements and yet the feelings we have for them are vital and part of what is most important in our lives. Most encounters with others contain the possible seeds of experiential knowledge. It is only when we are so detached from other people that we treat them as objects that no experiential learning can occur.

Not that all experiential knowledge is tied exclusively to relationships with other people. For example, I had considerable propositional knowledge about America before I went there. When I went there, all that propositional knowledge was changed considerably. What I had known was changed by my direct experience of the country. I had developed experiential knowledge of the place.

Experiential knowledge is necessarily personal and idiosyncratic. Indeed, as Rogers (1985) points out, it may be difficult to convey to another person in words. Words tend to be loaded with personal meanings and thus to understand each other we need to understand the nature of the way in which the people with whom we converse use words. It is arguable, however, that such experiential knowledge is sometimes conveyed to others through gesture, eye contact, tone of voice, inflection and all the other non-verbal and paralinguistic aspects of communication (Argyle 1975). Indeed, it may be experiential knowledge that is passed on when two people become very involved with each other in a conversation, a learning encounter or counselling.

As a development of the above discussion of three types of knowledge, it is possible to define experiential learning as any learning activity which enhances the development of experiential knowledge (Burnard 1987a). Experiential learning, then, is personal learning : learning that makes a difference to our self concept - a point developed by Knowles (1978, 1980) in his theory of andragogy, discussed below. As all interpersonal relationships with others, both within and without the health care professions involve an investment of self, it seems reasonable to argue that any learning methods that involve the self and that involve personal knowledge are likely to enhance personal effectiveness. We cannot, after all, learn interpersonal skills by rote, nor merely by mechanically learning a series of behaviours. We need to spend time reflecting on ourselves and on receiving feedback on our performance from other people.

The problem with the above discussion of experiential knowledge is this : how can we describe a domain of knowledge that we cannot clearly talk about or find words for? The weakness in any argument for a private and personal domain of knowledge within the person is two-fold. First, if such private thought worlds are inaccessible to others, we might ask how the **individual** accesses it. This raises the second problem of whether or not such private thought worlds are comprised of a "private language", peculiar to the individual in question. Again, the problem would seem to be one of access to it by the person or by others and also the translation of such a private language into the "public language" that we share with others. We would seem to have a least two choices here. Either we can abandon the notion of experiential knowledge and say, with Wittgenstein (1961 [1922]) that : "What we cannot speak about we must pass over in silence". Or we can stay with Polanyi (1958) in his argument that we "know more than we can say."

The particular characteristics of experiential learning

From the above discussion of experiential learning, from the theory of knowledge and from the historical perspective, it is possible to draw out those characteristics that go to make up the approach to learning known as experiential learning. It is not claimed that these characteristics are exhaustive of all aspects of experiential learning but they summarise aspects of experiential learning discussed in the literature.

In experiential learning there is an accent on action

Both the Dewey and the humanistic approaches to experiential learning involve the learner in action. This is not to say that the learner is "doing something" in a trivial sense but that she is engaged in an activity that should lead to learning. This is in opposition to traditional teaching/learning strategies which require that the learner remain passive in relation to an active teacher who is the dispenser of knowledge.

Freire (1972) called this traditional approach the "banking" approach to education : knowledge is delivered to the learner in chunks and the learner later cashes out this information in examinations. The experiential learning approach is closer to Freire's concept of "problem posing" education. Here, problems are encountered through discussion, argument and action. The learner is no longer passive but in dialogue with an equally active teacher. This characteristic is similar to the approach taken in Weil and McGill's, third "village" (above), with the accent on action and change.

There is a second, less important sense of action too. In experiential learning the learner is often physically moving to take part in structured activities, role play, psychodrama and so on, as opposed to more traditional learning situations in which the learner is seated behind a desk or table. These issues are discussed under the heading of **experiential learning methods**, below.

Learners are encouraged to reflect on their experience

Most writers acknowledge that experience alone is not sufficient to ensure that learning takes place. Importance is placed on the integration of new experience with past experience through the process of reflection (Kolb 1984, Kilty 1983, Freire 1972, Burnard 1985). Reflection may be an introspective act in which the learner alone integrates new experience with old. It may also be a group process whereby sense is made of an experience through group discussion.

23

A phenomenological approach is adopted by the facilitator

Phenomenology may be defined as the description of objects or situations without their being ascribed values, meanings or interpretations. Phenomenology as a philosophy was developed by Husserl (1931) and underpins the philosophical writings of the existentialists (Sartre 1956, Macquarrie 1972).

The facilitator who uses a phenomenological approach restricts himself to the use of description as a means of summarising what a learner has said and enables that learner to invest their her own learning with meaning. The "valuing" or "meaning" processes are left to the learner. It is the learner who ascribes meaning to what is going on in the learning environment and the facilitator's meanings are not automatically foisted on the student. Reflecting this phenomenological approach, which eschews interpretation of experience by another person, Carl Rogers (1983) prefers to use the term "facilitator of learning" rather than the more traditional terms "teacher" or "leader". In using such a descriptor he hoped to remove the connotation of the teacher as expert or authority in the interpretation of experience. In the literature on experiential learning, the term facilitator is often used in preference to the terms teacher, lecturer, tutor or leader. All this is in line with Weil and McGill's (1989) fourth "village" - that concerned with personal growth and development.

There is an accent on subjective human experience

Alfred North Whitehead (1933) discussed the problem of "dead knowledge" and asserted that knowledge kept no better than fish. The experiential approach to learning stresses the evolving, dynamic nature of knowledge. Rather than evoking R.S. Peters' (1972) concept of education as initiation into particular ways of knowing, it stresses the importance of the learner understanding and creating a view of the world in that learner's own terms. Postman and Weingartner (1969) noted that traditional education assumes a linear model of knowledge in which there is absolute truth and a single fixed reality. Citing anthropological evidence that our language tends to limit our view of reality (Worf 1955) and that the means by which subject matter is communicated fundamentally alters the content of that communication. Postman and Weingartner challenge the linear view of education, claiming that learners need to develop the ability to ask critical questions about any so-called "facts" that are presented to them.

Experiential learning allows for different means of communicating concepts, accounts for "multiple realities" and invites critical reflection. In this respect, it differs considerably from the traditional model of education and training.

Human experience is valued as a source of learning

The accent in experiential learning, through its variety of learning methods and through its name, is on experience. Learners are encouraged to reflect on past experiences to plan for future events. In formulating his concept of andragogy (the theory and practice of the education of adults), Malcolm Knowles (1978, 1980) stressed the value of experience in the sphere of adult learning. He maintained that as an individual matures so she accumulates an expanding reservoir of experience that causes her to become a rich resource for learning. Knowles argued that the resource should be tapped in the educational process because, as Knowles put it : "To an adult, his experience is who he is" (Knowles 1978). For Knowles, there was an important ontological issue : an adult's experience is not something exterior and tacked on but is part of the person's self-concept. Experiential learning then is an attempt to make use of human experience as part of the learning process. The humanistic approach to experiential learning pays particular attention to the emotional aspect of the individual's experience (Heron 1981). This approach is also typical of Weil and McGill's (1989) second "village', concerned as it is with adult learning theory.

The quest to define experiential learning exactly parallels the quest to develop a discrete theory of adult learning. The quest to develop a theory of adult learning has been a lengthy one. Kidd, writing in 1973 compared the search for such as theory to the search for Eldorado. Dubin and Okun (1973) and Lasker, Moore and Simpson (1980) suggest that individual learning styles are so idiosyncratic as to cast doubt on any general assertions as to how adults learn. Brookfield (1986) in a review of the literature on adult learning theories notes the ethnocentricity of much of the research in the field. He suggests that what research has been done has mostly been

25

concerned with white, American middle class learners. He poses the question :

> How can we write confidently of adult learning style in any generic sense when we know little (other than anecdotally) of the cognitive operations of, for example, Asian peasants, African tribespeople, or Chinese cooperative laborers? (Brookfield 1986 : 137)

This sort of question may help to keep in perspective the limitations of the general theories that have been developed about experiential learning, andragogy and other theories about how adults learn.

The literature on adult learning divides out into a few empirical studies aimed at trying to find out how adults learn and numerous theoretical papers about adult learning. In a way, the adult learning discipline is very similar to the discipline of nursing. In both, there tend to be more large scale theories than there are tightly constructed pieces of empirical work. The temptation in both fields is to develop ungrounded theory that rarely gets empirically tested. James (1983) reported the findings of a study into the basic principles of adult learning after a team of researchers had done a search of articles, research reports, dissertations and textbooks on adult learning.   Amongst other features, James reported the following principles of adult learning :

- adults maintain the ability to learn,
- adults are a highly diversified group of individuals,
- experience is a major resource in the learning situation,
- self-concept moves from dependency to independency as individuals grow in responsibility, experience and confidence,
- adults are motivated by a variety of factors,
- active learning participation in the learning process contributes to learning,
- a comfortable, supportive environment is a key to successful learning.

These principles were validated for James by an American jury of national adult education leaders and later validated further via a widely distributed questionnaire.

Andragogy

James' findings are very similar to the concepts discussed by Knowles under the heading of andragogy (Knowles 1980, 1984, Knowles and Associates 1984). Andragogy, a term associated with Knowles , though used before his time, was one used to differentiate the theory and practice of adult education from pedagogy – the theory and practice of the education of children. The assumptions in andragogy are four-fold and familiar to many nurse tutors. A truncated version of the four assumptions is as follows :

- Adults prefer to be self-directed in their learning projects,
- Adults' experience is a rich source of learning,
- Adults need to be able to **apply** what they learn,
- Adults' self-concept is affected by what they learn.

Whilst the principles of andragogy have been widely incorporated into the thinking and curriculum writing of nurse tutors, the concept of andragogy remains a controversial one. One objection that may be raised about Knowles' theory is that the ideas identified above may be applicable, also, to children. If this is the case, it is difficult to see how he can argue for a discreet theory of adult education based on these principles. Knowles acknowledges this problem and, in later writing, tends to describe andragogy as an attitude towards education rather than as being a discreet theory of adult education. This argument and others relating to andragogy have been well described by Jarvis (1983, 1984) and Brookfield (1987). Whilst Knowles has never claimed that his principles constitute an empirically based theory of adult learning, Jarvis notes that the theory of andragogy has

> acquired the status of an established doctrine in adult education, but without being grounded in sufficient empirical research to justify its dominant position (Jarvis 1984 : 65).

A number of reasons why andragogy has been so attractive to nurse tutors may be mooted. First, in its insistence on self-directedness and the development of self-image, it is in keeping with the humanistic approach to psychology and care. That humanistic approach, reaching a peak in mainstream psychology and education in the 1960's, came of age in nursing at a later date. The clearest statement of the call for a humanistic approach to nursing and nursing education came in the form of the 1982 syllabus of training for psychiatric nurses (ENB and WNB 1982). The humanistic approach remains an influence in more recent writings on nursing and nurse education (Vaughan and Pillmoor 1989, Riehl-Sisca 1989, Arnold and Boggs 1989, Jarvis and Gibson 1985). Another issue is that nurse educators seem, at last, to have acknowledged that people entering training do so as adults : perhaps this was not always the case. The recent interest in andragogy may demonstrate a shift in attitudes towards students by tutors : from seeing them as children to seeing them as adults.

Finally, whilst discussing the characteristics of experiential learning it may be noted that what is under consideration is :
a) a set of teaching/learning methods and
b) an attitude towards learning.

In the end, however, it is probably that the term "experiential learning" has almost limitless connotations. Henry (1989) in a study of 54 educators who responded to a questionnaire devised by that researcher found that the educators definitions of experiential learning were embraced by the following categories of learning methods and approaches :

- Independent learning,
- Personal development,
- Social change,
- Non-traditional learning,
- Prior learning,
- Work experience,
- Learning by doing,
- Problem-based learning.

Arguably, though, Henry's categories can be subsumed within one or more of the approaches to experiential learning outlined above:
- The Deweyian Approach,
- The Humanistic Psychology Approach,
- The "Four Villages" Approach.
- The Development of Experiential Knowledge,
- The Andragogical Approach.

28

Experiential Learning Methods

Experiential learning can also be viewed as a set of activity-based learning methods. In this section, methods that have been called "experiential learning methods" are reviewed as they relate to nurse training and education.

A wide variety of experiential learning methods have evolved out of the field of humanistic approach. All of those methods focus on the student or learner being offered an experience, followed by the reflection and making sense of that experience, as described in Kolb's learning cycle, outlined above. In this section, some of those methods are examined, critically for their use in interpersonal skills training and nurse education.

Pairs Exercises

Pairs exercises, are often advocated for use in the development of counselling and interpersonal skills in nursing and the health professions (Tschudin 1986, Heron 1983, Burnard 1989c, 1989d). The usual format for the pairs exercise is that each person nominates themselves "a" or "b". Then "a" practices the particular skill (for example, using open-ended questions) in the supportive presence of "B". After a period in these roles, the two people swap round and "b" practices the skill in the presence of "a". Afterwards, the group reforms and participants discuss their experiences.

An alternative use of the pairs format is for the pair in question to take a theme and for one person to discuss that theme whilst the other person listens. After a prescribed time, the pair switch roles and the listener becomes the talker and vice versa. After an equal amount of time in this second phase of the activity, the pair may link up with another pair and discuss the issue in a foursome. This method is called "snowballing" by Jarvis (1984)

Structured Group Activities

Structured group exercises allow for the experiential learning cycle to be worked through by a learning group. There are a number of publications describe a variety of group activities for enhancing interpersonal, social and counselling skills (Kagan, Evans and Kay 1986, Murgatroyd 1986, Burnard 1985). The idea of these activities is that the group undertakes an experience after which they discuss their thoughts and feelings about the experience and apply the new learning to the real or clinical situation. The adventures of this approach include the sharing of a common experience, the generation of a wide range of possible solutions to practical problems and the realisation of both the personal and the common nature of group experience.

Structured group activities as a form of experiential learning had been advocated by Marson (1979) as appropriate for the development of communication skills in nursing. Bailey (1983) writing of experiential learning techniques in psychiatric nurse training argued that structured group activities were geared towards uncovering unconscious material for expression and resolution in peer groups. This suggests, of course, that Bailey treated as unproblematic (at least in that paper) Freud's notion of "unconscious material" (Hall 1954) - an issue that has been highly criticised in recent times by Masson (1990) in his review of psychotherapy in general. Masson's view is that **all** forms of psychotherapy involve one set of values and beliefs (the therapist's) being imposed on another person (the client or patient). Also, Bailey's suggestion of the working out of "unconscious material" in an educational setting suggests a blending of education and therapy - an issue that will be returned to in the analysis of data in another chapter of this book. It may be noted, at this point, that various activities that have been adopted as experiential learning methods have their basis in forms of psychotherapy (role play, psychodrama and certain structured group activities).

Role Play

Role play involves the setting up of an imagined and possible situation, acting out that situation and learning from the drama (Figure 1.5) (Van Ments 1983, Argyle 1981, Dietrich 1978). More specifically, the cycle indicates that after a role play, a period of reflection is necessary, followed by feedback from other participants in order that new learning can be absorbed from the drama.

1. Setting the scene

2. Acting out the role play

3. Reflection and feedback

4. Integration of new learning from the role play

Figure 1.5 : The Stages Involved in Role-Play

The first stage of a successful role-play, "setting the scene", consists of inviting a number of participants to play out a scene, either from their own past or one they are likely to encounter in the future. Scenes replayed from the past are useful in that the role play allows further reflection on those past situations. Anticipated scenes, on the other hand, allow for the rehearsal of new behaviour

Once the "players" have been selected, scenery and props of a simple sort are used to create the invoked scene, for example, tables and chairs, suitably arranged.

Once scenery has been set and roles cast, the role play begins. The facilitator acts as "director" and helps the actors to fully exploit their roles. Occasionally the facilitator may stop the role play and allow a character to slow down her acting or take time out to consider how best to play the next part of the scene.

When the scene has been played out to the satisfaction of the players, the facilitator asks the players to reflect on their performances and those of their colleagues. Following a feedback period the role play can be re-run and new learning, gained from the feedback, can be incorporated into the new performance.

Role-play has been advocated for use in interpersonal skills training and in the development of counselling skills (Nelson-Jones 1981, Burnard 1989d), group facilitation skills (Heron 1989a), assertiveness skills (Alberti and Emmons 1982) and social skills (Ellis and Whittington 1981).

Apart from the use of role play in the development of interpersonal skills, it may also be used as an aid to developing empathy; to rehearse initial practitioner/client meetings; to develop interview skills; to practice public speaking or the delivery of seminar papers and as a problem-solving activity. In this later context, a problem situation is acted out with a variety of possible "solutions". The actors and the audience decide which solution feels best after they have completed the various role-plays. Richardson, Bishop,

Caygill et al (1990) described an extended form of role play in which mental handicap nursing students were encouraged to play the part of profoundly dependent patients for a period of 24 hours, in order to attempt to experience empathy with such patients.

Role play has been widely advocated for use in the training of nurses and as an example of an experiential learning activity in the nursing education literature (Wibley 1983, Heath 1983, Barnes 1983, McNulty 1984, Kilty 1983, Dietrich, 1978, Goble 1990).

Psychodrama

A variant of role play is psychodrama (Moreno 1959, 1969,1977, Blatner 1988) In psychodrama, a "real life" situation that has been lived by one or more of the group members is re-enacted and then discussed by those actors and by the group. The above stages are worked through in psychodrama in much the same ways as they are in standard role-play. Slight variations in approach may be noted, however, and the following stages offer a more complete guide to the process of psychodrama:

1. the scene to be replayed is selected,

2. the main "actor", who has described the scene to be re-enacted, chooses fellow actors, from the group, to play other parts,

3. the main actor briefs those actors about their roles and gives them a clear outline of what happened in the real situation.

4. the psychodrama scene is played out. As it is, the main actor may stop the action to suggest small changes in performance. The aim is to, as completely as possible, recreate the past scene.

5. the performance is then processed by the group of actors and ideas are offered by any "onlookers".

6. after the discussion, the situation is replayed as the main actors would have liked it to have occurred.

Again, psychodrama has been advocated for encouraging the development of assertiveness and counselling skills and communication skills (Siegel and Scipio-Skinner 1983, Reed 1984). Watkins and Addison (1990) described an extended version of psychodrama as a form or theatre for encouraging nurses to explore their relationships with patients. It has also been used for exploring group members personal and professional life problems (Gonen 1971, Rowan and Dryden 1989). Both psychodrama and role play can invoke considerable emotion in both players and observers (Logan 1971).

The founder of psychodrama, Moreno, was a charismatic person. Clare (1981) noted the numerous reports of Moreno's charismatic qualities and the dramatic and overwhelming qualities of trained psychodrama therapists. Clare concluded that :

> In therapy after therapy, from est to primal therapy, TA to Gestalt, one encounters the difficulty in distinguishing between faith in the therapist and evidence that the therapy actually works, that is to say, that it produces in the final analysis what it promises. (Clare 1981 : 109).

This issue, the question of whether or not therapies (and indeed dramatic experiential learning activities) are carried out by charismatic people whose charismatic influence is, perhaps, as influential as the therapy or educational experience, itself, is an interesting and fraught one that we shall return to again in the analysis of data later in this book.

Goble (1990) after reviewing the literature on psychodrama advocated its use as an experiential learning activity for the development of interpersonal skills in nurse education programmes. He also identified some differences between role play and psychodrama in terms of purpose, focus, emotional content,scenarios enacted and duration of activity (Fig. 1.6)

	ROLE PLAY	PSYCHODRAMA
Purpose	Training	Therapy
Focus	Professional	Personal
Emotional Content	Low	High
Scenarios Enacted	Usually future work situations	Private life : distant past/ present/ future
Duration of Activity	Usually less than 15 minutes	Up to three hours

Figure 1.6 : Summary of the Major Differences Between Role Play and Psychodrama (After Goble 1990)

Experiential Learning in Interpersonal Skills Training in Nursing

In the past two decades, there has been an increasing interest in the development of interpersonal skills in nursing. Interpersonal skills have been defined by Kagan (1985) as :

> ...those aspects of both communication and social skills that are concerned with **direct person-to-person contact.**
> (Kagan 1985 : 1)

A variety of studies have been carried out in the field of interpersonal skills in nursing. Early studies tended to focus on patient satisfaction surveys (McGee 1961, Hugh-Jones, Tanser and Whitby 1964, Ley 1972). Later, observation studies that described and analysed nurse-patient interaction were carried out (Altschul 1972, Cormack 1976, Norton, McLaren and Exton-Smith 1976) and in more recent times there have been studies of the effectiveness of teaching interpersonal skills to nurses (Jasmin and Hill 1978, Fielding 1983). Jasmin and Hill found that video taped recordings of nurses' interpersonal performance was a means of encouraging self-awareness in nurses.

Fielding's (1983) study also explored the implications of video taping in the increase of nurse's awareness of their communication skills. Macleod Clark (1985) noted that most of the educational methods under review in such studies can be described as "experiential" and that such methods are not easy to assess objectively. It is asserted, here, that the questions raised in the present study are also an attempt to clarify the field : we cannot assess the effectiveness of experiential learning and experiential learning methods until we identify what they are.

Interpersonal skills in nursing have been variously described. Arnold and Boggs (1989) include the skills of developing and structuring nurse-patient relationships, organising and running group activities and coping with partings (such as following bereavement). Ellis and Watson (1987) describe the development of communication skills as part of interpersonal skills development in nursing. Burnard (1990) has suggested that basic counselling and group facilitation skills are other aspects of the field of interpersonal skills in nursing. Tschudin (1986) and Kenworthy and Nicklin (1989) also describe the need for nurses to develop counselling skills as part of interpersonal skills training programmes. Various interpersonal skills training programmes for nurses have also been described in psychiatric nursing (Reynolds 1985, Reynolds and Cormack 1987) and general nursing (Marshfield 1985, Raichura, 1987).

Experiential learning methods have been advocated for use in teaching interpersonal skills to nurses. Ellis and Watson (1987) describe the use of group therapy techniques as a form of experiential learning in the development of communication skills. Role play has been recommended as a method of teaching social skills to nurses by Ellis and Whittington (1981). Various books of experiential learning exercises for interpersonal skills development in nurses have also appeared (Kagan, Evans and Kay 1986, Burnard 1989c, 1990, Kilty 1983, Arnold and Boggs 1989, Porritt 1990)

Conclusion

The field of experiential learning is broad and diverse. It encompasses a number of overlapping and yet differing aspects. On the one hand it has been described as a process of learning from experience, either through the process of living or by the setting up of a variety of possible experiences by a teacher or therapist. On the other hand, it has been described as a series of particular sorts of activities : role play, psychodrama, structured group activities and so forth. Experiential learning activities have been advocated for helping to develop interpersonal skills in nursing students and also for the training of psychiatric nurses. It is the diversity of the term "experiential learning" that has made research in the field so difficult to date.

No doubt, this variety of definition and description is the case in other fields. It is not assumed that the term "experiential learning" is any clearer in other health care settings nor, generally, in secondary, further and higher education. Whether or not it is important to continue to clarify terms is open to some debate. What was notable in the study described in this book was that students and tutors did not necessarily perceive the same sorts of things when they were subject to experiential learning. Nor did either group necessarily define and describe experiential learning in the same sorts of terms. If educational activities are to be clear and understood by both students and teachers, it would seem to be important that the question of educational nomenclature be addressed.

2 Studying experiential learning

This chapter identifies the design and methodology of a study which explored the nature of experiential learning with tutors and students. It includes the following sections :
* The aim of the study,
* An overview of the research design,
* A discussion of the qualitative and quantitative research methods in the social sciences.

Introduction

The previous chapter discussed the literature as it relates to experiential learning and experiential learning methods. This chapter outlines the design of the present study and offers a discussion of some of the factors that determined the way in which the study was planned and executed.

Aim of the Study

The aim of this study was to explore nurse tutors' and students' perceptions of experiential learning in order to develop both theoretical and practical models of experiential learning for practice. This aim was to be achieved through the use of two approaches : semi-structured interviews of small groups of nurse tutors and students, followed by the development of a questionnaire to be used to survey a larger sample of nurse tutors and students.

Before specific details of the research plan are described, some theoretical issues directly related to this style and method of researching are discussed.

Overview of the Research Design

The methodology used in this study was dictated by the nature of the research aim (Bogdan and Biklen 1982, Field and Morse 1985). Having elected to explore people's perceptions of experiential learning, qualitative, factor searching research methods were required.

The descriptors, phenomenological and grounded theory may both be used to describe the general approach used in the first part of this study. These are forms of qualitative research and as such aim to develop theory inductively (Field and Morse 1985, Glaser and Strauss 1967).

Phenomenology attempts to describe a situation stripped of preconditions, values or beliefs. Oiler (1982) suggests that phenomenology represents the effort to describe human experience as it is lived. Its origins can be found in the work of the existential writers, particularly Husserl (1931) but also Heidegger, Merleau-Ponty, and Sartre, (Patka 1972, Macquarrie 1972). In this study, the aim was not to start out with a particular set of beliefs or theories about experiential learning (though, clearly, the researcher had these), but to examine and explore the beliefs and theories of others, whilst attempting to "bracket" the researchers own beliefs and theories (Husserl 1931). The notion of bracketing refers to the putting on one side of any value judgements that one might have about the subject in hand. Husserl argued that such a process of investigation lead to a clearer perception of the matter under investigation. The degree to which it is possible to bracket one's own beliefs and theories remains open to question.

If it **were** possible to engage in this bracketing process completely, then the researcher would be working in a theoretical void, with no means of making sense of what the respondents were saying nor any means of knowing how to proceed. Nevertheless, the attempt has been made to ensure that the researcher's own beliefs and theories colour the material to a minimal degree. Following Reason and Rowan (1981) the researcher wrote a paper outlining his own beliefs and values about the subject area before commencing work on the research project. A summary of some of the points in that paper has been included as part of the introduction to this book. The aim of such an enterprise is to bring to consciousness those beliefs and values that may affect future work. Simon, Howe and Kirschenbaum (1978) refer to this process as values clarification.

Two other methods were employed to attempt to cut down bias on the part of the researcher. One was a conscious effort on the part of the researcher to constantly check his own tendency to "lead" in an interview or to rush to interpret the data that were collected. By "interpret", here, is meant any attempt to prejudge how the other person was using words or to "make sense" of what they were saying in terms of a particular theory. Here, we run into linguistic problems and problems of "personal" versus "shared" meanings. On the one hand, we cannot suppose that other people are using words in a way that corresponds to a dictionary definition or a technical definition. As Wittgenstein (1961) pointed out "meaning is use" : when a person uses a word, he does so according to what he believes it to mean. There is no guarantee that the meaning that he imputes corresponds to the meaning imputed by the listener.

On the other hand, if there was no occasion on which shared meanings were possible, we could not communicate with one another, for every word spoken by an individual would acquire a "personal" meaning that was not comprehensible to another person. A sense of how this could feel can be gained when a person who speaks another language to our own (and which we do not understand) begins to talk to us in that language. Clearly, communication is considerably impaired. The only time, in such a situation, that we can guess at what the person is talking about is when he uses a word that sounds similar to a word in our own language. In that case, we guess at meaning, in order to try to make sense of what he is saying. So it is, to a degree, in everyday conversation. We are constantly (and metaphorically) asking the question : "what does he mean?" If we cannot answer the question to our own satisfaction then we will find ourselves confused and unable to make sense of the conversation. Clearly, such a state of affairs calls for a theory of "shared" as well as "personal" meanings.

This, then, is the problem of shared versus individual meaning. The method employed in this study to attempt to deal with this issue was to frequently check with the respondent what they meant by a particular word that they used. Hinkle (1965) suggests that "laddering" or the frequent use of "why?" questions can help in this respect. This approach was occasionally used but a more frequent approach was to simply ask the respondent to explain how he was using a particular word. It is acknowledged that such an approach is hardly foolproof. Clearly, to ask a person, after the event, what he meant by a particular word is no guarantee that the definition that he offers captures the full sense of usage. To ponder on the meaning of a word or expression after we have used it may lead us to expand on our thoughts about that word or expression. It is possible, too, that we do not always know what we mean when we use some words. Sometimes we get to understand the meanings of words by using them first, by "trying them out", in order to explore how we could use them in the future.

The second method used to attempt to check any tendency on the part of the researcher to colour data with his own meaning and belief system was to frequently check any analysis that was carried out with the respondent. Later on in this report I will describe how, once an interview had been analysed, that analysis was discussed with the respondent to further check for clarity and for the capturing of individual meaning. It is asserted that this is in line with the phenomenological approach to research.

Grounded theory is a deductive approach to exploring and developing a theory of what is happening in a given situation. The basic principles of the approach were developed by Glaser and Strauss (1967) who suggested that, for too long, social scientists had tended towards the development of "grand theories" that were not necessarily grounded in what was happening in the world. In other words, social scientists had tended to adopt a deductive approach : first they developed a theory about the social world and then they set out to test the degree to which that theory could be held to be true. Inevitably, argued Glasser and Strauss, the temptation (consciously or unconsciously) was to confirm and develop the prepared theory. They suggest, therefore, that the opposite approach be adopted : that the social scientist first goes out and explores an aspect of the social

40

world, immerses himself in it and allows himself to discover what is there. Only after this immersion has taken place do they recommend that theory about the social world be developed and then that the theory should be firmly grounded in the data obtained : hence "grounded theory".

Glaser and Strauss, having spelt out their objections to traditional approaches to social science research are then less specific about how the grounded theory approach should be operationalised. A number of research studies (Pollock 1989, Melia 1986) suggest that those studies were carried out "in the spirit of grounded theory". Other commentators have criticised Glaser and Strauss' lack of clarity (Stern 1985) and given this disparity between the criticism of traditional research techniques and their description of how the problem may be rectified may lead to questions about the degree to which the grounded theory approach represents a discrete research methodology at all. It could be argued that the approach represents a prescription about how to do certain sorts of research, without that prescription having been fully worked out. This may not invalidate Glasser and Strauss' criticisms of deductive approaches to research but the issue of whether or not it is possible to do "pure" grounded theory research remains an interesting question as does the degree to which grounded theory can be completely differentiated from other sorts of phenomenological and qualitative approaches. The question of whether or not there is a need to draw such definite lines between concepts may be answered by considering that if we cannot clearly say what the grounded theory approach is and how it can be operationalised, then we are likely to run into problems in, at least, the following areas : defending grounded theory as a research approach at all, addressing questions of validity and reliability, using the approach in practice, developing theory out of the collected data.

Qualitative and Quantitative Methods in Social Science Research

There is considerable discussion in the literature about whether or not the differences between qualitative and quantitative methodologies are differences of fundamental philosophies or whether they are differences of method (see, for example the reviews in Bryman 1988, Leininger 1985, Van Maanen 1983). At the philosophical level it is argued that the quantitative researcher adopts the position of determinism : that the world is always and everywhere subject to

41

causal laws (Bullock and Stallybrass 1977). If causality is a "fact" about the world, then the way to explore that world scientifically is to collect, measure and count examples of things that happen in it as a means of developing theories and laws. On the other hand, the qualitative researcher seems to be arguing that our perception of what happens in the world is always dependent on a number of variables that colour our perception of it (for example, our physiological make up, our cultural context, our education, our belief systems and so on) : thus we cannot ever perceive the world "as it is" but only "as we believe it to be".

Therefore, the idea that we can ever cleanly and objectively collect, measure and count examples of things that happen in the world in order to develop laws and theories is always problematic. The qualitative researcher therefore tends to adopt a relativistic position and denies the validity of the quantitative researchers' position. It remains an open question as to whether all researchers question the philosophical bases that their methods rest upon but it may be argued that our beliefs and theories about the way the world is will always fuel our actions. Indeed, Claxton, seems to be attempting to bridge the philosophical differences between the absolutism of the extreme quantitative position and the relativism of the extreme qualitative position when he suggests that,

> What I do depends on what my theory tells me about the
> world, not on how the world really is, (and)... What
> happens next depends on how the world really is, not on
> how I believe it to be. (Claxton 1984 : 17).

At first glance, Claxton's position seems to echo that of the theorists who argue that everything is relative and that we can, as William James would have it, only observe the phenomena, never the noumena (James 1902). Caxton, however, goes further than this in suggesting that the world "really is" a certain way and that we can somehow make comparisons between what we believe to be true and what is actually true. This begs questions about how it is possible to know that the world "really is" a certain way (for Caxton to posit the idea that the world "really is" a certain way is to suggest certainty that the world "really is" a certain way. Another position would be that the world may be a certain way but it may not "be" any particular way at all). Caxton seems to want to have an absolutist world working away beneath the surface of our theories and beliefs about it. If he is right, then he may offer a key to a marriage between quantitative and qualitative methods.

If there are, indeed, two things happening : a world as it actually is and people in it that are viewing it and theorising about it, it would seem reasonable to combine both quantitative and qualitative methodologies. On the one hand, the quantitative methods offer a systematic way of classifying and quantifying the world, as accurately as possible. On the other hand, the qualitative methods offer a means of studying peoples belief and meaning systems. Thus, the argument is often developed that a combination of the two methods should be used. It is this position that is adopted in this study : both quantitative and qualitative methods are used, although the predominant method is qualitative. It is not intended that the differences between the two approaches (in practice) be rehearsed here · those differences have been explored in detail in the considerable literature on the topic (see, for example Cook and Reichardt 1979, Filstead 1970, Gaut 1984, Pelto 1970, Raggucci 1972 and Van Maanen 1983).

In summary, then, the researcher set out to both explore individuals' perceptions of experiential learning (the qualitative aspect) and also to identify whether or not there was some agreement over the ways in which experiential learning was perceived by groups of people (the quantitative aspect). In a sense, no research project can ever be purely qualitative : every qualitative researcher necessarily engages in some form of categorisation and quantification in order to present his findings. The only way of getting close to "pure" qualitative research would be to present raw data and to allow the reader to make sense of it. Even if this dubious practice was engaged in, the reader would presumably then begin his own categorisation and quantification processes.

Price and Barrell (1980) and Barrell, Medeiros and Barrell (1985) offer precedents for the approach taken in this research project. They suggest moving from personal views of the world (in this case, via qualitative analyses of interviews) through to larger scale investigations to identify any tendency towards consensus of otherwise (in this case, via questionnaires to identify the degree to which the perceptions of those interviewed are or are not the perceptions held by a larger group of people).

3 Perceptions of experiential learning

This chapter describes the first part of the data collection and analyses in the research study. It explores the following issues :

- The sample,
- Ethical issues,
- Access to the sample,
- The interview method,
- Methods of analyses of the interviews.

Introduction

The chapter describes the first stage of the study in which interviews were carried out to explore a small group of nurse tutors' and student nurses' perceptions of experiential learning.

Sample

First, it was decided to interview a group of 12 nurse tutors regarding their views of experiential learning. The criterion for inclusion in this group was that the nurse educator claimed to be using experiential learning methods in his/her work with student nurses. Following Bogdan and Taylor's (1982) suggestion about obtaining respondents, the researcher often asked the person who was being interviewed to recommend another person whom that respondent knew to be using experiential learning methods. This has also been called the snowballing approach to selecting a sample (Field and Morse 1985). Thus a purposive sample (Fink and Kosecoff 1985) emerged. Bogdan and Biklen (1982) describe such a sample as one which is designed to best facilitate the emergence of relevant theory.

The sample of tutors was made up of a variety of nurse tutors from England and Wales (and one from Australia) working in both general and psychiatric nursing. All claimed to use experiential learning methods in their educational practice. Whilst no differences between psychiatric nurse teachers and general nurse teachers was looked for nor elicited, a future study may usefully look at possible differences. The sample included lecturers (3), senior tutors (2) and nurse tutors (7).

The sample of student nurses was a convenience one. A convenience sample is one in which respondents are approached because they are available to talk and because of limitations of time. The students invited to take part were all students who worked in some of the hospitals in which the nurse tutors worked. A convenience sample was used because of the impossibility of random sampling and because no credible list of criteria could be drawn up for selecting **particular** students. The aim of this part of the study was to explore a number of student's perceptions of experiential learning. As no statistical analysis was to be carried out on the data obtained and because no generalisation of the findings (without further research) was to be engaged in, all that was required was that some students who were prepared to talk about their perceptions of experiential learning would be approached. All students who were asked if they would be prepared to be interviewed did so voluntarily and no student approached refused to take part. As the students were all working at hospitals in which the tutors worked, it was (correctly) assumed that all had taken part in what were described by their tutors as "experiential learning activities".

Ethical Clearance

In some health authorities, it is a requirement that all research proposals be presented to an ethics committee for approval (Burnard and Chapman 1988). In the areas from which data was obtained, ethical approval only had to be sought if patients were to be interviewed (although this situation had changed by the time the researcher came to distribute a questionnaire). As patients were not being approached in this study, no such application had to be made in order to carry out the first stage of the project (although ethical clearance **was** required for part of the second stage of the project and that is discussed below).

Gaining Access

Whilst Bogdan and Taylor (1982) suggest that access to respondents should be obtained by whatever means possible, other writers on research methods suggest that access should be obtained formally (Kidder and Judd 1986, Youngman 1978). The aim of requesting access to respondents formally is that it ensures that everyone concerned with the study is fully aware of the researcher's presence and that the researcher is obtaining data with the respondents' (and their superior's) informed consent. To this end, access to both tutors and students was gained by seeking and obtaining permission via a series of letters down the professional hierarchy. Thus, in the first instance, The Director of Nurse Education, in each hospital was contacted, then the senior tutors and then the individual tutors. In no case was access denied and in no case did anyone refuse to be interviewed. In each case, each respondent was told of the aim of the research, in keeping with Reason and Rowan's (1981) and Jourard's (1964) suggestion that researchers in the social sciences should be open about their intentions.

Interview Method

The interview was chosen as the method of exploring the tutors' and students' perceptions. The semi-structured interview method was the main tool used (Spradley 1979). This means that whilst certain topics

46

were nearly always referred to in each interview (eg. definitions, evaluation methods), the order in which these topics were talked about was dictated more by the way in which the interview developed than by prior planning on the part of the interviewer. During the interview, the broad, open question was the question of choice (Heron 1989b, Egan 1990). Broad, open questions are those that allow the respondent considerable latitude in the way they both interpret and choose to answer the question. An example of such a question would be "What are your thoughts about evaluating experiential learning?" This is deemed preferable to closed questions (eg "Do you evaluate experiential learning?") or to more specific open questions ("How do you evaluate experiential learning?") as they allow the respondent greater freedom to express his own thoughts and beliefs about the topic under discussion and no sense of "leading" is likely to be experienood.

During the interview, a range of client-centred counselling responses were used by the researcher, ranging from reflection (echoing the last few words used by the respondent, back to the respondent) (Rogers 1951, Heron 1989b, Egan 1990), through to "minimal prompts" ("yes", "go on" etc.) Heron (1989b) describes these sorts of interventions as catalytic and suggests that they encourage the respondent to develop a particular line of thinking without the interviewer adding to or subtracting from what is going on. Such an approach is also in keeping with the phenomenological and grounded theory approaches referred to above, in that they represent an attempt to enter the perceptual world of the other person without attempting to influence or lead that person.

Whilst client-centred counselling methods were employed, the researcher was keenly aware that a research interview differs in important ways from a counselling interview in that the aims and intentions of the persons carrying out research and counselling will be different. The general approach to talking to people is similar in both settings. Carl Rogers, founder of client-centred therapy (Rogers 1961, 1967, 1983) has often been described as adopting a phenomenological approach to counselling (Hilgard and Atkinson 1982, Nye 1986). One of the aims in both client-centred counselling and in phenomenological research is to explore the perceptual world of the other person. In counselling, this leads to a therapeutic end. In research it leads to a process of clarification and theory development.

The advantages of this method are : the content of the interview can dictate the direction that the rest of the interview takes; the researcher can invite the interviewee to expand and develop a particular theme; the relationship that exists between the interviewer and interviewee can enhance the clarification and development of the interviewee's thinking and verbalising (Douglas 1985). The disadvantages of the approach include the following : the data that emerge are non-standard in that each interview may differ in its content and structure, thus making analysis more difficult; the interviewer may "lead" the interviewee in certain ways, thus intentionally or unintentionally influencing what the subject says. On balance, however, it was decided that the interview method had distinct advantages over the questionnaire in that it was more flexible and could be more readily adapted to identify respondents' meaning systems than could the questionnaire.

A semi-structured interview schedule was constructed and piloted in two ways. First, the researcher asked a colleague to play the role of an interviewee and to play "devil"s advocate" (Heron 1982) and to raise any doubts at all about the style and content of the interview. This proved to be a useful method of clarifying certain types of questioning technique and of helping to ensure that no ambiguities were present in the questions to be asked.

Second, the interview schedule was used with two tutors who were not part of the study. The resulting interviews were not transcribed but listened to directly from the tape recordings made. Following these two trial runs, the interview schedule was again modified slightly. One of the problems of using the semi -structured approach is that a set list of questions is not used, therefore the pilot study can never be an exact trial run for subsequent interviews as any interviews that followed would necessarily be different to those carried out during the piloting. On the other hand, such piloting did allow for ambiguities in questioning to be acknowledged and corrected and tendencies for "leading" the interviewee to be modified.

Interviews with nurse tutors were then carried out that lasted for between 30 and 45 minutes each. The student nurse interviews ran for the same time. The interviews were taped for later transcription. All respondents were asked for their permission for the interviews to be taped and no one refused.

After some experimentation with recording devices, it was decided that an ordinary household cassette player would be used to record the interviews. This was one of the researchers' children's "ghetto blasters" which, being a stereo cassette player and recorder, has a microphone at each end of a fairly lengthy "body" and is also battery powered. This was placed between the researcher and respondent and proved to be a very satisfactory means of taping interviews. Also, it is asserted that such an "everyday" item may help the interviewer to relax more quickly than would be the case if more "technical" equipment was used or it both researcher and respondent were required to wear neck microphones.

Following taping, each interview was transcribed. This was carried out by the researcher typing directly onto a wordprocessing program on a computer, using the "pause" button on the tape recorder to stop after small passages of the recording had been played. Everything that both researcher and respondent said was written down in this way and three full stops were used to indicate a pause by either party (...). As the researcher transcribed, he was able to get a deeper and closer "feel" for the data and made notes on sheets of paper next to the computer regarding themes and categories emerging as he transcribed. He also wrote down any thoughts and feelings that occurred to him as he worked. This is in keeping with Bogdan and Biklens' (1982) suggestion that copious field notes are useful to any researcher working with qualitative data. Not all of the notes were later used but they proved useful in clarifying passages of the text on further readings and in helping the researcher to develop the category systems described in the final sections of this chapter.

The process of transcription is an extremely time-consuming one. Although the researcher is a touch typist, he estimated that one hour of interview took approximately five hours to transcribe. The possibility of asking other persons to transcribe was considered but in the end the decision to self-transcribe was taken because of the perceived advantage of "indwelling" within the data that this transcription encouraged.

Analyses of the Interviews

Two methods of analysis were used in order to approach the data in two different ways. In the first instance, a simple content analysis of the interview transcripts was carried out in order to begin to get a feel for the general themes that were under discussion. This type of analysis was combined with a frequency count of the occurrence of the categories noted in the data and this is presented in tabular form. In the second form of analysis a more detailed, more qualitative approach was adopted in order to get a comprehensive picture of the respondents' perceptions.

The same methods of analysis were used for both the tutors' and the students' interviews.

Initial Analysis

First, a content analysis (Carney 1972, Lofland 1971, Berg 1989) was performed on the transcripts. Such a method of analysis aims only at identifying the overt content of interviews : it cannot hope to identify latent content (Fox 1982). Overt content refers to the meanings in written or spoken data that are clear and unequivocal : no attempt is made to look for hidden meanings (Babbie 1979). Latent content refers to hidden or personal meanings that are usually present in all speech and writing and yet which are extremely difficult to access during data analysis.

Initially, all the transcripts were read through and then categories were identified from the questions that had been asked. The broad category headings that emerged from the tutors' interviews, for example, were :

● Definitions of experiential learning,
● Examples of experiential learning methods,
● Examples of learning methods other than experiential learning methods,
● Advantages of the experiential learning approach
● Disadvantages of the experiential learning approach,
● Evaluation methods.

The transcripts were then re-read to determine what each of the interviewees had said under each of the headings. In this way, a series of sub headings was generated from the data. During this process a number of categories were "collapsed" to form clearer, more discrete sets of categories. Reliability checks were undertaken by inviting a colleague to read through a number of transcripts and to identify her perception of the categories. Agreement was then reached on "core" categories.

Using these sub headings it was then possible to read through the transcripts again and note to what degree there was agreement or disagreement about definitions, methods and so forth, between the interviewees. A grid was drawn up which showed the categories and sub categories (Field and Morse 1985). An example of part of that grid is illustrated in Figure 3.1. Each transcript was reexamined and the presence or absence of an interviewees' response to a particular category or subcategory was noted.

No limitation was placed on the number of subcategories that could be identified within a particular category from a particular transcript.

DEFINITIONS

	Learning from past experience	Learning from present experience	Whole life experience
Interviewee 1	X		
Interviewee 2			X
Interviewee 3		X	

Figure 3.1 Example from the analytical grid

Validity

The question of the validity of this categorisation process was considered. If, as Glaser and Strauss (1967) suggest, the aim of ethnomethodological and phenomenological research is to offer a glimpse of another person's perceptual world, then the researcher should attempt to offset his own bias and subjectivity that must creep through any attempt at making sense of interview data. Two methods of checking for validity were used in this stage of the study. First, the researcher asked a colleague who was not involved in any other

51

aspect of the study but who was familiar with the process of category generation in the style of Glaser and Strauss, to read through three transcripts and to identify a category system. The categories generated in this way were then discussed with the researcher and compared with the researcher's own category system. The two category analyses proved to be very similar which suggests at least three possibilities :

a) the original category analysis was reasonably complete and accurate,

b) the original category analysis was too broad and general in nature and thus easily identified and corroborated by another person,

c) the colleague was anticipating the sorts of categories that the researcher may have found and offering the researcher "what he wanted to hear".

The last possibility can be reasonably ruled out on the grounds that the colleague was unfamiliar with both the subject and content of the present study prior to being asked to help validate the category system and, as a recently employed member of the department, was unaware of the researchers' own work and research interests.

The question of whether or not the category system was too broad and general in nature may be countered by the fact that the original system had been developed by a "funnelling" process : many categories were generated at first and these were then distilled down to a smaller number by the process of "collapsing", described above. It is to be hoped, therefore, that the agreement of both parties over the category system helps to suggest that the system had some internal validity.

The second check for validity was that of returning to three of the people interviewed and asking them to read through the transcripts of their interviews and asking them to jot down what they saw as the main points that emerged from the interview. This produced a list of headings which were then compared with the researcher's and the two lists were discussed with the respondents. Out of these discussions, minor adjustments were made to the category system, although, (as with the first method of validating the category system), the two lists of headings and categories were very similar. Another method of checking the validity of this research project is described at the end of chapter 7.

Following the generation and validation of categories in this way, each category was given an identifying number and all of the interviews were coded in the manner suggested by Strauss (1986) and

Field and Morse (1986). Thus, each transcript was read through and the corresponding code placed in the margins of the transcript to indicate that here was an example of the category. In this way it was possible to account for nearly all of the data in the transcripts.

Once the coding process was complete, the coded sections of the interview transcripts were cut out and pasted together in order that a complete collection of coded items could be collected together under each category. In this way, it was possible to scan through all of the data that had been collected within a given category and to make minor adjustments to ensure that a good fit was achieved between coded items and categories.   At this stage, too, a further check for validity was carried out. One of the people interviewed was approached and the categorising and coding of her interview was discussed with her to identify whether or not she felt that the categorisation and coding of her interview transcript captured the essence of what she had said and what she had meant. There are numerous problems here. First of all, the subject is being asked to review material drawn from her interview but presented in a different order to the original presentation. This may render the original material difficult to identify. Second, the subject is being asked to reconsider what she has said some months after she has said it. The fact that the researcher is present and asking the subject to consider the validity of his work, is likely to put pressure on the subject to agree with or approve the researcher's work. On the hand, gross distortion of what a person has said is likely to be noticeable to that person and thus the method of checking for validity seems to be a reasonable, further check for validity.

In the situation described here, the subject agreed that the analysis into categories represented a fair description of what had been discussed in the interview.

Secondary Analysis

A modified grounded theory approach was used for the secondary analysis, to explore the latent content of the interview transcripts (Glaser and Strauss 1967). The grounded theory approach offers a means of searching for "emerging" themes and categories from research data which are then developed into "theories". This is the opposite way round to most traditional research methods which tend to start with an assumption and then seek to identify whether or not that assumption is true. The grounded theory approach starts from a naive, naturalistic position. The researcher is asked to attempt to start researching without any prior assumptions about the subject matter or field of enquiry. The degree to which this is possible, is debatable.

It is important to state in what ways this aspect of the project was **not** a true grounded theory study. First, the topic under consideration – experiential learning – had already been written about, described and discussed in some detail in the literature. Therefore the research was not addressing an "unknown" field. Grounded theory is usually used to explore uncharted territory. Second, the method known as "constant comparative analysis" (Glaser and Strauss 1967), whereby each interview transcript was compared with the previous one in order to modify future interviews was not adhered to. In **this** study, the aim was to explore each person's perceptions of experiential learning in order to develop a fairly detailed picture of the scene prior to developing a questionnaire for a larger survey.

The Method of Secondary Analysis

The method was developed out of those described in the grounded theory literature (Glasser and Strauss 1964, Strauss 1982) and in the literature on content analysis (Fox 1982, Babbie 1979, Couchman and Dawson 1990) and out of other sources concerned with the analysis of qualitative data (Field and Morse 1985, Bryman 1988).

Aim of the Analysis

To produce a detailed and systematic recording of the themes and issues addressed in the interviews and to link the themes and interviews together under a reasonably exhaustive category system. This was achieved by the rigourous working through of the interview transcripts, the use of "open coding", the "collapsing" of overlapping categories and the final production of a category system that accounted for almost all of the issues that had been discussed by the respondents. In this way, the categories can be said to have "emerged" from the data in the style of the grounded theory approach.

In any analysis of qualitative data there is the problem of what to **leave out** of an analysis of a transcript. Ideally, all of the data should be accounted for under a category or sub category (Glaser and Strauss 1967). In practice there are always elements of interviews that are unusable in an analysis. Field and Morse (1985) refer to this data as "dross". In order to illustrate what was **not** included in the analysis of the interviews presently under discussion, it may be helpful to offer an example of data that were considered not to be categorisable nor considered to add to the general understanding of the field under consideration.

> "I don't know, like they say, now they say it was alright, whereas before, perhaps, you wouldn't."

Whilst the person in this example is trying to convey something it would be difficult to know what it was. As an aside to this discussion, it is interesting to note that such "uncodable" pieces of transcript only appear to be unusable at the analysis stage. During the interviews, all of what was being said appeared to be quite coherent to the researcher.

In the next four chapters, the findings from the interview data are identified and discussed. Chapters 4 and 5 identify the findings from the **initial** analyses. Chapter 6 and 7 identify those from the **secondary** analyses.

4 Tutors' perceptions of experiential learning: Part one

In this chapter the findings from the initial analysis of the tutors' interviews are described.

Categories

The broad categories that emerged out of the initial analysis of the tutors' interviews were :

- Definitions of experiential learning,
- Examples of experiential learning methods,
- Examples of learning methods other than experiential learning methods,
- Advantages of the experiential learning approach
- Disadvantages of the experiential learning approach,
- Evaluation methods.

Definitions

The first category identified in the part of the study was that of definitions of experiential learning. Table 4.1 illustrates the subcategories that were generated from the transcripts, along with the frequency with which they were cited by the tutors and placed in rank order.

Table 4.1

Definitions of Experiential Learning (n = 12)

DEFINITIONS	FREQUENCY
1. Learning through doing	8
2. Affective learning	4
3. Whole life experience	4
4. Learning from past experience	3
5. Learning from present experience	3
6. Role play	1

A range of definitions was offered - there was no general agreement about what constituted experiential learning. The range varied from the most frequently cited definition (learning through doing) to definitions which accented various dimensions of life experience: the whole of life, past life experience and present life experience - the "here and now". One interviewee saw experiential learning as being synonymous with role play : an interesting finding, since more usually role play is seen as an example of an experiential learning method rather than as a definition (see the section below, on methods).

Some of the interviewees admitted that they found experiential learning difficult to define. This is a curious statement given that all of the respondents claimed to be using experiential learning methods in their day-to-day teaching, and had acknowledged a strong interest in the concept prior to the research. If they are using it extensively, then it is not too much to expect them to be clear in their own minds about what it is and how it works. This paradox may suggest a limitation in the method used in the study. Perhaps a period of observation in the learning environment with some of the nurse tutors and students could help to clarify the situation.

The variety of ways of defining experiential learning is interesting in that it suggests that it may be defined by different people in different sorts of ways. If nurse tutors vary in their definitions of experiential learning it seems likely that learners will perceive experiential learning in different ways. On the other hand, it is difficult to know to what degree differences of definition are important as there was much less difference of opinion about what constituted experiential learning methods (see the next section).

Experiential Learning Methods

The next category to be identified was that of experiential learning methods. Interviewees were asked to identify what they would describe as examples of experiential learning methods. Table 4.2 illustrates the sub categories that were generated in this section.

Table 4.2
Examples of Experiential Learning Methods (n = 12)

EXPERIENTIAL LEARNING METHODS	FREQUENCY
1. Reflective activities	9
2. Role play	8
3. Practical activities	7
4. Structured group activities	5
5. Humanistic therapies	3
6. Games and simulations	3
7. Altered states of consciousness	2
8. Learning machines	2
9. Physical activities	2

A majority of those interviewed identified activities that involved reflection on experience as being examples of experiential learning methods. Some identified role play as a method, whilst others talked of practical activities such as getting learner nurses to feed each other or practising making beds with the learners as "patients". Some also described structured group activities of the sort described by Pfeiffer and Jones (1974 and ongoing) as examples of experiential learning methods. These usually involved the group undertaking a well defined activity in the group, followed by a period of reflection and sharing of the experience. A number of respondents also referred to a wide range of humanistic therapies as examples of experiential

58

learning methods. These included transactional analysis, gestalt therapy, co-counselling and encounter group work (Shaffer 1978).

A small number of those interviewed referred to methods that involved altered states of consciousness including meditation, trance work and Neuro-Linguistic Programming (Bandler and Grinder 1979). Others referred to games and simulations as examples of experiential learning methods. Only two referred to the use of videos or T.V.'s as examples and two referred to physical activities that involved active movement on the part of the learners. These examples were perhaps less diverse in their range than had been the definitions of experiential learning and the methods cited by the interviewees were supported by the literature on experiential learning which tends to refer consistently to role play, structured activities and a range of "therapeutic" activities (see, for example Kilty 1983, Burnard 1985, Heron 1973)

Thus a broad range of definitions but a narrow band of methods emerged as a consistent trend. As we noted above, perhaps the fact that there is considerable agreement on the things that may be called experiential learning methods is more important, from a practical, educational point of view, than is the diversity of opinion over definitions of experiential learning. On the other hand, it may be that tutors and lecturers have taken on board the popular "buzz words and phrases" in nurse education, without too much thought or consideration about how these new ideas may affect their teaching practice. If this latter scenario is at all accurate, then the outlook for developing more caring and interpersonally skilled nurses in the future is far from promising.

What is not clear from this analysis is the degree to which the tutors distinguish between educational activities and therapeutic activities. There may or may not be a contractual issue here : learners may come to an educational enterprise expecting to receive education. It would appear that some may receive "therapy", in the form of the "humanistic therapies" identified above or in terms of altered states of consciousness. The distinction between education and therapy clearly deserves greater clarification.

Comparison with other learning methods

When they discussed examples of learning methods other than experiential learning methods, the most frequently cited method was the lecture method. Other interviewees identified "teacher-centred" methods: seminars, reading and watching videos. Again, this is in keeping with the literature on experiential and allied learning approaches and particularly, perhaps with the student-centred approach of the late humanistic educator and psychotherapist, Carl Rogers (1983), who stressed the need to avoid teacher centred methods and lecturing in order to maximise learning from experience. The aim of this particular question was to identify a contrasting method with which the experiential learning approach could be compared.

Advantages of the Experiential Learning Approach

Interviewees identified what they perceived as being the advantages of the experiential learning approach. Table 4.3 illustrates the range of ideas generated in this area.

The most frequently referred to advantages of the approach were that they were useful for teaching interpersonal skills and that they increased self-awareness. These points are reinforced by the literature on the topic (Kagan 1985, Kagan et al 1986), although the concept of "self-awareness" remains problematic and none of the interviewees offered clear definitions of what self-awareness was. Some of the interviewees referred to concepts such as "real", "whole" or "active" as descriptors of the advantages of experiential learning. These are necessarily difficult to classify and perhaps to define. Only two of those interviewed saw experiential learning methods as advantageous in the teaching of practical nursing skills.

Some saw them as being lighthearted or fun to use, whilst two saw them as being more relaxed in their approach than with other types of methods and one person identified them as being easier to use than other methods. The "other" methods, here, refers to more traditional lecture and teacher-centred approaches.

Table 4.3
Advantages of the Experiential Learning Approach (n = 12)

ADVANTAGES	FREQUENCY
1. Useful for teaching interpersonal skills.	5
2. Experiential learning increases self-awareness.	
3. "Real"/"whole"/"active".	5
4. Lighthearted/fun.	4
5. Tutor enjoys using them.	3
6. More relaxed than other methods.	2
7. Useful for teaching practical nursing	2
skills.	2
8. Easier to use than other methods.	1

Interviewees discussed the disadvantages of the approach. Table 4.4 shows the sub categories generated in this area. A majority of those interviewed acknowledged that learners undertaking experiential learning may find it uncomfortable or threatening. Many felt that this was because experiential learning was a more "personal" approach to learning as opposed to the more impersonal lecture method. As we have noted, above, a limitation of this type of analysis is that it refers only to the overt content of the interview transcripts.

Table 4.4
Disadvantages of the Experiential Learning Approach
(n = 12)

DISADVANTAGES	FREQUENCY
1. Can be uncomfortable/threatening for the learners	9
2. Not suitable for all topics on the syllabus	5
3. Need lots of planning	4
4. Time consuming	3
5. Transfer of learning may be a problem	1

It would be interesting to explore the latent content in this particular area. It may tentatively be hypobooked, for instance, that some of the discomfort and threat identified in this section may be projected discomfort and threat, on the part of the tutors. In other words, the perceived discomfort may have been an expression of the educator's own discomfort. This must remain conjecture, however, for the method of analysis does not allow for this type of hypobook to be tested.

However, the mention of threat and discomfort is again intriguing. Why would advocates of a particular approach, which incidentally is much more positive and encouraging in style than the traditional methods of learning, continue to use a mode of teaching which is disliked by the learners? Where is the negotiated curriculum and the encouragement for the learner to have a say? These and similar questions may be answered in some part by the next stage of analysis.

Some suggested that a disadvantage may be that experiential learning was not suitable for all topics on the timetable, it is interesting and perhaps paradoxical that others had identified experiential learning (above, under definitions) as involving the whole of life experience. Further, it is perhaps, reasonable to expect that no one method will be suitable for learning or teaching all topics on a curriculum. The need to engage in lots of planning was identified as a disadvantage by four people, three found experiential learning time consuming and one was concerned with the issue of whether or not the learning gained from an experiential learning session carried over into the "real" situation (the "transfer of learning" problem). This issue has been discussed in more detail in the increasing literature on clinical teaching and ward-based training (Marson 1979, Ogier 1982, Fretwell 1982).

Evaluating Experiential Learning

The interviewees also talked about how they evaluated experiential learning. Table 4.5 outlines sub categories generated in this area. The most frequently cited method of evaluating experiential learning was to ask the learners to feedback their opinion of the usefulness or value of the experience at the end of an experiential learning session. This method is frequently cited in the literature on experiential learning (Kilty 1982, 1984, Burnard 1985, Heron 1973) although, arguably it allows only a very subjective "impressionistic" picture of learning to emerge. Also, it anticipates that learning can be evaluated so soon after the experience. It is arguable that other evaluation methods need to be used after some time has elapsed and in order for full assimilation of the learning to take place (Clift and Imrie 1981). Some of those interviewed said that they asked for written evaluation reports from their students and a minority used repertory grid techniques (Bannister and Fransella 1986). One said that she asked for reports from nurses working on the wards and used these as an indicator of the effectiveness or otherwise of experiential learning and one said that she observed the learners on the wards to evaluate them in a similar way. A number of the interviewees noted that evaluation of experiential learning was "difficult". The subjective nature of experiential learning must continue to make the subject of evaluation an awkward one.

Table 4.5

Evaluation Methods in Experiential Learning (n = 12)

EVALUATION METHODS	FREQUENCY
1. Verbal feedback from the group	10
2. Written reports from students	5
3. Repertory grid techniques	2
4. Reports from the ward	1
5. Observation	1

5 Students' perceptions of experiential learning: Part one

In this chapter the findings from the intial analysis of the students interviews are described.

Method of Analysis and Categories

The method used to undertake the initial analysis of the students' interview transcripts matched the process used to analyse the tutors'. A different set of categories emerged in this analysis, otherwise the process was the same as with the tutors' interviews.   The broad category headings that were used were as follows:
- Definitions of experiential learning,
- Experiential learning activities used in the school of nursing,
- Experiential learning in clinical settings,
- Advantages of the experiential learning activities used in the school of nursing,
- Disadvantages of the experiential learning activities used in the school of nursing,

A difference in emphasis could be noted in the students' responses when compared to those of the tutors. The students tended to distinguish between experiential learning as a form of **clinical** learning and experiential learning as a set of methods or activities used in the school or college of nursing. Whilst some of the tutors had alluded to the notion of experiential learning covering learning in the clinical setting, the distinction was not so marked as to warrant a separate category for it in the analytical framework. Notably, though, when the students came to discuss the advantages and disadvantages of the experiential learning approach, they tended to discuss those methods and activities used in the school of nursing. This may have been due to at least two possibilities. Reading through the researcher's questioning in these interviews, it is noticeable that there was a tendency for issues concerning the "school version" of experiential learning to be discussed more than the "clinical version". Also, it is possible that interviewees expected that the interviewer was exploring **school** based experiential learning. One respondent suggested to the researcher that :

"If you're doing some research into experiential learning, I suppose it's something to do with comparing experiential learning with traditional methods of teaching."

The implication, here, seems to be that the respondent perceives the researcher to be doing research about **teaching** methods. Also, all of the respondents knew that the researcher was a lecturer in nursing in a university. All of this may have added to the tendency for both respondents and researcher to concentrate on the **school** aspects of experiential learning. In future research, however, it would be useful to clarify this position and to explore both clinical and school approaches more equally.

Definitions of Experiential Learning

The students' responses to the issue of what experiential learning was are illustrated in table 5.1. It will be noted that most described experiential learning in terms of it being concerned with learning through doing. This was linked, closely, with the notion of it concerning "practice" rather than "theory" and with a negative definition of experiential learning as it **not** being "textbook learning".

A number of the students volunteered that they perceived experiential learning as a series of exercises and activities used in the school or college of nursing, although almost the same number saw it as learning in the clinical setting. This issue did not arise when **tutors** offered definitions of experiential learning. Notably, too, the tutors sometimes saw experiential learning as being concerned with the education of the affect, or to do with the emotional side of nursing education, whilst this was not an issue pursued by the students.

Some students also defined experiential learning negatively as "not being "chalk and talk" " - or not being traditional methods of teaching and learning. Some also took a middle path and saw experiential learning as combining elements of both clinical and school learning. One student referred to experiential learning as concerning the whole of life experience, whilst this was more frequently described by the nurse tutors.

Table 5.1
Definitions of Experiential Learning (n = 12)

DEFINITIONS	FREQUENCY
1. Learning through doing	10
2. "Practice" rather than "theory"	9
3. Not textbook learning	9
4. Exercises used in the school or college of nursing	8
5. Learning in the clinical setting	7
6. Not "talk and chalk" learning	2
7. School learning and clinical learning combined	2
8. Whole of life experience	1

Experiential Learning Activities in the School or College of Nursing

As we have noted, the students tended to make a distinction between experiential learning as something taking place in the clinical setting and experiential learning as a series of exercises or activities in which they took part in the school or college of nursing. Table 5.2. illustrates the sorts of activities described by the students as ones they had taken part in.

All but one of the students had experienced taking part in role play, whilst this had been number two in the tutors' list of activities. A number of students described their taking part in counselling skills activities and four had been involved in psychodrama. The following activities were described by three students : the "blind walk" exercise, small group exercises, empathy building activities and the practising of practical nursing skills. The "blind walk" activity is one in which students are blindfolded and led around by a colleague. The activity has been described as having various purposes, such as its use as a "getting to know you" activity (Kilty 1983) and as the means of exploring visual deprivation (Burnard 1985).

Empathy building activities are discussed and described by Rogers (1967) and Egan (1990) as methods for encouraging students to enter another person's frame of reference. The term "small group activity" could easily cover a range of educational activities and is not a particularly specific descriptor although it is notable that such a category arose in the analysis of the tutors' transcripts. The type of activity that stands out as different to the others in this category is the "practising of practical nursing skills". Three students described how they were encouraged to practice such skills both in the school or college of nursing and in the clinical setting by ward managers. Whilst those students identified this as an experiential learning method, the nurse tutors did not.

A minority described their taking part in "icebreakers" or "warm-up" activities. Again, these activities are widely described in the literature as methods of helping a learning group to relax and to prepare for an interactive group learning session (Heron 1982, Burnard 1990).

Table 5.2
Experiential Learning Activities
Taken Part in the School or College of Nursing (n = 12)

EXPERIENTIAL LEARNING ACTIVITIES TAKEN PART IN THE SCHOOL OR COLLEGE OF NURSING	FREQUENCY
1. Role play	11
2. Counselling skills exercises	6
3. Psychodrama	4
4. "Blind walk" exercise	3
5. Small group activities	3
6. Empathy building exercises	3
7. Practising practical nursing skills	3
8. Icebreakers	2

Experiential Learning in the Clinical Setting

As noted above, the students who were interviewed identified the **clinical area** as an aspect of experiential learning. Table 5.3. illustrates the issues identified under this heading. Most felt that working in the clinical areas offered them a valuable source of learning about nursing and most felt that clinical work was more valuable as a learning resource than learning from books. This helps to reinforce the notion referred to by **both** groups of interviewees : experiential learning as learning by doing. What was noticeable, though, was that this issue was more emphasised by the students than by the tutors.

Some students felt that learning in the clinical setting was more "real" than learning in the classroom or school of nursing, although this issue was not developed in any of the interviews. Finally, in this section, 5 of the students acknowledged that school learning and clinical learning are not always linked and a minority of those interviewed felt that tutors tended to get out of touch with the clinical setting.

Table 5.3
Experiential Learning in Clinical Settings (n = 12)

EXPERIENTIAL LEARNING IN CLINICAL SETTINGS	FREQUENCY
1. Clinical work is a valuable source of learning	9
2. Clinical work is more valuable a learning resource than "textbook" learning	8
3. Clinical learning is "real"	7
4. Learning in the school or college of nursing and clinical learning are not always linked	5

Advantages of the Experiential Learning Approach

The other issues that were identified in the first analysis of the students' interviews related to the use of experiential learning methods and activities used in the school or college of nursing. Sometimes the school or college aspect of experiential learning was returned to by the student herself and sometimes the researcher developed that aspect of the interview. With hindsight, it would have been preferable for the interviewer to have also developed the issue of clinical work as a form of experiential learning.

The three most commonly cited advantages of the experiential learning approaches used in the school or nursing, as perceived by the students, echoed very closely the perceptions of the tutors (Table 5.4). Eight of the students felt that experiential learning activities gave them the chance to learn directly from personal experience, further emphasising the "learning by doing" approach. The same number felt that experiential learning methods helped them to develop interpersonal skills but did not elaborate as to how this may be the case, except to note that they had been encouraged to practice counselling and listening skills. Eight also offered the more general view that experiential learning methods were a general aid to learning.

Six of the students felt that experiential learning activities were fun to take part in, thus echoing and complementing some of the educator's who said that they enjoyed using them. This would be in line with Rogers' (1983) idea that a learning environment in which both learners and teachers are relaxed and enjoying learning is more likely to be a productive one than the converse. Finally, in this section,

69

four students noted that experiential learning methods encouraged reflection on what they were doing both in the school of nursing and in their work as nurses in the clinical or community settings.

Table 5.4
Advantages of the Use of
Experiential Learning Activities
Used in the School or College of Nursing (n = 12)

ADVANTAGES OF THE USE OF EXPERIENTIAL LEARNING ACTIVITIES USED IN THE SCHOOL OR COLLEGE OF NURSING	FREQUENCY
1. They give you the chance to learn from personal experience	8
2. They help you to develop interpersonal skills	8
3. They are a general aid to learning	8
4. They are enjoyable	6
5. They encourage reflection	4

Disadvantages of the Experiential Learning Approach

The two most frequently cited disadvantages of the experiential learning approach used in the school or college was that such approaches were "unreal" and that they did not suit all learners (Table 5.5). These were not issues raised by the nurse tutors who worried more that experiential learning methods may be uncomfortable or threatening for the learners. Indeed, 5 of the students referred to the idea that those methods may be threatening and the same number also felt that some experiential learning methods could be embarrassing to take part in. Four went further and described some of the learning methods that they had taken part in as "silly". Three acknowledged that they didn't like role play. Finally, the idea that experiential learning methods could get out of control was mentioned by one respondent as was the fact that the experiential learning activities used in one school of nursing always seemed to cover the same ground ; notably the development of basic listening and counselling skills.

70

Table 5.5

Disadvantages of the Use of Experiential Learning Activities Used in the School or College of Nursing (n = 12)

DISADVANTAGES OF THE USE OF EXPERIENTIAL LEARNING ACTIVITIES USED IN THE SCHOOL OR COLLEGE OF NURSING	FREQUENCY
1. They are unreal	7
2. They don't suit all learners	7
3. They can be threatening	5
4. They can be embarrassing	5
5. They can be silly	4
6. I don't like role play	3
7. They could get out of control	1
8. The activities always cover the same ground	1

Comparisons : Tutors' and Students' Perceptions of Experiential Learning

From this initial content analysis of the transcripts of both tutors' and students' interviews it became apparent that there were at least four areas of overlap in the types of distinctions that both groups made when discussing experiential learning. Those areas were :

● Definitions of experiential learning,
● Experiential learning methods,
● Advantages of the use of experiential learning methods,
● Disadvantages of the use of experiential learning methods.

That is not to say that each group always identified the same points under each of those headings but merely to note the general areas of similarity in discussion. Beyond those two areas of similarity, two points of divergence were noted. First, the students tended to discuss experiential learning more in terms of **clinical work** than did the tutors. Second, the tutors discussed methods of **evaluating** experiential learning, whilst the students did not.

A number of explanations may be offered for these initial findings. First, on the issue of the students' discussing clinical work as a form of experiential learning, it can be noted that students spend more of their working lives in the clinical setting than they do in the school of nursing. Conversely, the tutors tend to work most often in the schools or colleges of nursing. On the other hand, the difference in perceptions may also point to the theory-practice gap that has been identified in other studies and in the literature. It could be the case that the students tended to see their primary source of learning about nursing as the clinical, rather than the school, setting. This idea is further supported by their description of clinical work as being more "real" and of the experiential learning activities carried out in the school of nursing as "unreal". "Reality" it would seem, for the students, is working in the ward or the community.

On the issue of evaluating experiential learning, it is unsurprising that the nurse tutors tended to discuss this as an issue given that much of the literature on teaching and learning stresses the importance of evaluating learning and teaching (see, for example : Kenworthy and Nicklin 1989, Jarvis 1987, Minton 1984). It is less likely, however, that students will have reviewed this literature or place such a high value on evaluation and assessment of learning.

In the final part of this chapter, the comparisons between the tutors' and students' perceptions of experiential learning are explored.

Comparison One : Definitions

First, both groups tended most often to define experiential learning in terms of "learning by doing". The student group seemed to reinforce this practical issue in their descriptions of experiential learning being "practice rather than theory" and in their negative definition of experiential learning as "not textbook learning" and "not chalk and talk". On the other hand, the tutors tended to emphasise the **affective** element in experiential learning and to discuss experiential learning as learning that involved personal and life experience. Whilst experiential learning was often viewed as involving the whole of life experience by the tutors, it was less frequently seen in this way by the students.

In general, it seems that the students linked experiential learning far more specifically to the job of doing nursing and learning about nursing in the clinical setting than did the tutors. Meanwhile the tutors tended to take a more "personalised" view of the process, seeing it as the means by which all sorts of aspects of a person's

experience were brought to the learning arena. Table 5.6. summarises
the differences between the two groups on the issue of definition.

Table 5.6
Comparisons : Tutors and Students :
Definitions of Experiential Learning

DEFINITIONS OF EXPERIENTIAL LEARNING

TUTORS	STUDENTS
1. Learning through doing	1. Learning through doing
2. Affective learning	2. "Practice" rather than "theory"
3. Whole life experience	3. Not textbook learning
4. Learning from past experience	4. Exercises used in the school or college of nursing
5. Learning from present experience	5. Learning in the clinical setting
6. Role play	6. Not "talk and chalk" learning
	7. School learning and clinical learning combined
	8. Whole of life experience

Comparison Two : Methods

When it came to discussing experiential learning methods there were
less noticeable differences between the two groups. Both discussed a
range of activities ranging from role play to various sorts of small
group activities. Some of the tutors were more specific about the
sorts of exercises and activities that they used and linked them to
particulary theoretical bases (eg humanistic psychology). This was the
case with the students. Again, this is perhaps unsuprising given that
the literature on experiential learning often has links with the
humanistic psychology literature (see, for example Heron 1989b,
Burnard 1990). Also, it seems less likely that students will have read
educational literature of this sort given that their primary focus of
learning in nursing.

One noticeable difference between the priorities of the two groups is that although both identify role play as a prime example of experiential learning methods, the tutors identify **reflective activities** prior to discussing role play. This may be linked to the increasing discussion in the nursing education literature about the "reflective practitioner" and for the need for nurses to reflect on what they do (Schon 1983, Boud et al 1985). The literature on experiential learning often refers to the process of reflecting on experience (Kolb 1984, Kagan, Evans and Kay 1986, Heron 1973).

Table 5.6 summarises the differences between the two groups on the issue of definitions of experiential learning.

What seemed to be emerging at this point was a distinction between **experiential learning** as a philosophy, an approach, an attitude towards learning, on the one hand, and **experiential learning methods** as a group of learning activities, methods or exercises on the other. Whilst both groups had taken part in or used experiential learning methods in their education or educational practice, **experiential learning** was far more difficult to pin down and define. Table 5.7 summarises the differences between the two groups on the issue of experiential learning methods.

Table 5.7
Comparisons : Tutors and Students :
Experiential Learning Methods

EXPERIENTIAL LEARNING METHODS

TUTORS	STUDENTS
1. Reflective activities	1. Role play
2. Role play	2. Counselling skills exercises
3. Practical activities	3. Psychodrama
4. Structured group activities	4. "Blind walk" exercise
5. Humanistic therapies	5. Small group activities
6. Games and simulations	6. Empathy building exercises
7. Altered states of consciousness	7. Practising practical nursing skills
8. Learning machines	8. Icebreakers
9. Physical activities	

Comparison Three : Perceived Advantages

The key issues of similarity between the two groups under the heading of advantages appeared to be that experiential learning methods encouraged the development of interpersonal skills, they drew on personal experience and were enjoyable to take part in. The students identified the issue of reflection on experience that was discussed, above, by the tutors.

Whilst the literature on interpersonal skills training (counselling skills, talking and listening, running groups, communicating with patients etc) has frequently recommended the use of experiential learning methods in recent years (Kagan, Evans and Kay 1986, Burnard 1989c, Heron 1982, Kilty 1983), that literature is nearly always **prescriptive** in nature and whilst recommending experiential learning methods as appropriate for teaching and learning interpersonal skills does not offer empirical evidence for the effectiveness of such methods.

On the issue of experiential learning methods being enjoyable to take part in, Rogers (1983) suggests that learning is enhanced when students enjoy the learning process and feel comfortable in the learning encounter. On the other hand, there seems to be no evidence for the idea that enjoyment of the process is a necessary condition for learning. Whilst it may be argued that students (and possibly teachers) are more likely to enjoy their education if they are enjoying learning sessions, it seems quite possible that people also learn under conditions of stress and anxiety - particularly in emergencies (Atkinson, Atkinson, Smith, et al 1990). Table 5.8 summarises the differences between the two groups on the issue of the perceived advantages of experiential learning methods.

Table 5.8
Comparisons : Tutors and Students :
Perceived Advantages of the
Use of Experiential Learning Methods

ADVANTAGES OF THE USE OF EXPERIENTIAL
LEARNING METHODS

TUTORS	STUDENTS
1. Useful for teaching interpersonal skills.	1. They give you the chance to learn from personal experience
2. Experiential learning increases self-awareness.	2. They help you to develop interpersonal skills
3."Real"/"whole"/"active".	3. They are a general aid to learning
4. Lighthearted/fun.	4. They are enjoyable
5. Tutor enjoys using them.	5. They encourage reflection
6. More relaxed than other methods.	
7. Useful for teaching practical nursing skills.	
8. Easier to use than other methods.	

Comparison Four : Perceived Disadvantages

Developing the theme, discussed above, of whether or not the learning experience should be enjoyable, both groups identified that one of the disadvantages of experiential learning methods are that they could be threatening or uncomfortable for the learner. Again, this seems to support a view that the learning process should be a pleasant and comfortable one rather than a threatening one. A number of writers in the educational field have stressed the need for challenging students through critical dialogue and of the need for such challenge as a means of pushing the students on the question their own beliefs, values and attitudes (Postman and Weingartner 1969, Brookfield 1986, 1987, Jarvis 1987).

On the other hand, Jarvis (1983) has also stressed the need for the process of adult education to honour the dignity of the learner and some of the students identified that experiential learning methods could be embarrassing and "silly" and that such activities could get "out of control". Table 5.9 summarises the differences between the two groups on the issue of the perceived disadvantages of experiential learning methods.

Table 5.9
Comparisons : Tutors and Students :
Perceived Disadvantages of the
Use of Experiential Learning Methods

DISADVANTAGES OF THE USE OF EXPERIENTIAL
LEARNING METHODS

TUTORS	STUDENTS
1. Can be uncomfortable / threatening for the learners,	1. They are unreal,
	2. They don't suit all learners,
	3. They can be threatening,
	4. They can be embarrassing,
2. Not suitable for all topics on the syllabus,	5. They can be silly,
	6. I don't like role play,
	7. They could get out of control,
3. Need lots of planning,	8. The activities always cover the same ground.
4. Time consuming,	
5. Transfer of learning may be a problem.	

These are some of the points of comparison between the responses of the tutors and of the students. In later chapters, following further analysis and the survey of larger samples, many of these issues will be returned to. In the next chapter, the findings of the **secondary** analysis of the tutors' interviews are identified.

6 Tutors' perceptions of experiential learning: Part two

This chapter describes the findings from the secondary analysis of the tutors' interviews, as described in chapter three.

The Nurse Tutors' Perceptions

The following categories and sub categories emerged from this analysis :

1. Defining the Field

a) definitions of experiential learning,
b) experiential learning in clinical practice
c) experiential learning methods
d) Teaching/learning methods that are NOT experiential learning methods

2. Theories About Experiential Learning

a) Theories about learning,
b) Theories about experiential learning
c) Theories about the nature of personal experience
d) Theories about student choice in learning
e) Therapy and experiential learning
f) Emotions and experiential learning
g) Self awareness

3. Using Experiential Learning Methods

a) Rationale for using experiential learning and experiential learning methods
b) Using experiential learning methods
c) Students' responses
d) Evaluation of experiential learning
e) Advantages of experiential learning
f) Disadvantages of experiential learning
g) Learning to use experiential learning methods
h) Influences

The ordering of the categories in these sections was decided upon by examining all of the categories and looking for patterns and groups of categories. An initial category "system" was thus devised as a means of presenting the findings. As always, in qualitative and phenomenological research, the aim was to offer an honest and understandable presentation of the data in a format that illuminated the respondent's thoughts, ideas and meaning systems without adding to, nor subtracting from them (Parlett 1981).

In the presentation of findings, below, each of the categories and sub categories is discussed in relation to the literature on the particular topic, where this is appropriate. The aim of this approach is to begin to build up a picture of "what is" for the respondents with "what is in the literature". Again, this approach has been used by Glasser and Strauss (1967) and more recently (and in a nursing context) by Melia (1984).

Defining the Field

In order to begin to understand how nurse tutors understood the concept of experiential learning, it was useful to explore their methods of defining terms. In the first section, it is noted how they defined the expression "experiential learning". Such definitions were sometimes offered by the tutors' as a response to a question such as "how would you define experiential learning?" At other times, the definition emerged during the interview as a means of the educator making clear how he or she used that term.

In the second section, the nurse tutors described what they would count as "experiential learning methods". Again, sometimes this was in response to a direct request by the researcher for examples of experiential learning methods. At other times, the tutors' offered examples to illuminate what they were discussing or as a means of describing their practice.

In the final section of this first part, the educator's descriptions of what count as negative examples. That is to say that they suggest methods and approaches that they would not call experiential. This method of offering negative examples is a useful means of describing the boundaries of a concept.

Definitions of Experiential Learning

Very often, the first attempts an educator made at defining experiential learning proved tautological. Clear examples of this are as follows:

"I think it is learning from experience..."

"I look upon it as experiencing things..."

"Experiential learning is learning from experience..."

Such definitions were often followed by a more detailed account of how the educator perceived experiential learning. Sometimes, however, there were clearly problems in verbalising definitions :

"To me, experiential activity can be non-descriptive in the sense that people allow things to happen and then

you can discuss what has happened without...
prediscussion... I think anything can be turned to an
experiential level..."

The educator, here, appears to have been struggling to put into
words something that may have been clear to him. On the other hand,
the example may point to the idea that we do not always work with
"definitions" in our everyday lives. If we were to ask the person in the
street to define "music", it is probable that he or she would have
difficulty in doing so, though most people "know" what music is.
Indeed, the person may try to define music through offering examples
of "pieces of music". So, later on, we will note that many of the nurse
tutors were able to offer examples of experiential learning **methods**
as examples of what they were talking about, whilst finding formal
definition of the topic difficult. There may be something artificial in
asking people to define terms formally. This idea is supported by
some of the tutors' difficulty in defining experiential learning :

"I think it is difficult to define and I would say that it is
concerned with learning that occurs at the present time,
in the here - and - now, as they say..."

"I think it is very difficult to define. I can't think of a
precise definition of it but I always look on it as
actually doing things, experiencing things..."

This difficulty in definition may have been fuelled by another
factor : as we have noted in the literature, the term "experiential
learning" is often defined loosely and its definition may vary from
author to author in important ways. As we noted, some writers
(Knowles 1978, Keeton 1982) use the term to cover a range of
activities in which the learner has considerable choice over what he
or she does or what he or she learns. Other writers, notable those
from the humanistic school emphasise the accent on personal,
subjective experience. We will see, below, that the humanist influence
has apparently been felt by some nurse tutors.
Whilst some tutors defined experiential learning
tautologically and others had difficulty in defining it, others, still,
used all-encompassing definitions:

"I think any activity could be experiential..."

"I suppose using the term experiential could involve anything..."

The problem with such an all-encompassing approach is that it leaves open the question as to whether or not the term means anything at all. If experiential learning can involve "anything" then it may not be particularly useful to have such a term : it becomes superfluous. On the other hand, it was clear that even those people who described experiential learning in such broad terms had in mind **something** when they discussed experiential learning in as much as they went on to compare and contrast it with other sorts of things. Again, it is possible that asking people to define terms in a fairly formal way is problematic.

For some, the accent in defining experiential learning was on a time factor. Examples of this time dimension include

"Learning about things by doing it and also by learning from the past. Ploughing through your previous experience and reflecting on that and then using what you can get from it to go forward."

Although this respondent's insistence on moving forward is not all that clearly argued, he seems to be suggesting a pattern on learning from past experience which is echoed in Kolb's experiential learning cycle, discussed earlier. For Kolb, an important aspect of learning from experience is the ability to reflect on that experience as a means of gleaning guidelines for the future. This idea of learning from the past and relating it to the present is echoed by another respondent who said that:

"...Its learning from past experience as well as present experience."

and another who said:

"So I suppose its learning from experiencing something at the present time. Or maybe even in the future."

This respondent, however, did not dwell upon a theory of HOW a person may learn from experiencing something at the present time,

83

though the notion of forward movement in time is present again. Sometimes, the accent was more definitely on the present.

> "It (experiential learning) has to be here - and - now...for me..."

> "I would say that it is concerned with learning that occurs at the present time, in the here - and - now, as they say."

This accent on the here - and - now, on present time, is reflected in the humanistic literature on the topic of learning. Humanistic psychology, drawing as it does, from existentialism, often emphasises the need for people to pay attention to what is happening to them in the here and now as a means of personal development, therapy or even as a way of living (Rowan 1988, Shaffer 1978).

The argument behind this position can be spelt out as follows. All that we have "exists" in the present. The past is just that (and likely to be remembered inaccurately). The future has yet to occur. Thus the only time that we can be fairly sure about is our existence in the present. For the humanistic therapist and educator, the accent on the present is a crucial one. Given that existentialism as a personal philosophy accents the person's inherent capacity to choose and decide for himself (Sartre 1955, Pakta 1972), then such decision making can only take place with any certainty if we are fully aware of the present. To "live in the past" is to act with Sartrian (Sartre 1955) "bad faith" (or to deny one's full responsibility for choosing and deciding for one's self). To live in the future (in the sense of always anticipating something else) is, again, less than ideal as such prediction of the future is unlikely to be accurate. For the existentialist, then, the "place to live" is the present.

The tutors who discussed experiential learning in terms of "the here - and - now" appear to be supporting this notion of living in present time and linking teaching and educating with such an idea. This is congruent with Knowles (1978, 1985) concept of **andragogy** or the theory and practice of the education of adults. Knowles argues, amongst other things, that adults cannot afford to undertake "deferred learning". He suggests, by way of contrast, that children often have to learn things that will not be of immediate use or which will not have immediate application. He suggests that, for adults, **applicability** is essential. Adults, because of their appreciation of the passing of

84

time, usually choose not to engage in learning things that they will not use until later. Instead, they prefer to learn things that they will be able to use and which apply to their present, everyday life.

This practical aspect of learning through present time experience is developed by another of the tutors:

> "So for me (experiential learning) meant things like the clinical placement of student nurses in wards for experience : the practical aspect of nursing that they get in the ward placements, because they were doing things from which they were learning from. But I think the notion of experiential learning extends beyond just the practical "doing" things. I think it also involves anything that one experiences : a) practically, from the point of doing things or b) it is at a psychic level where in conversation with other people, or in contact with other people, relationships with other people - working experience also comes into it. So, if you like, it is a question of learning from those things which we all do."

Here, the respondent seems to emphasise the practical, utility value of experiential learning as a tool for teaching and learning nursing. He also seems to be hinting at a more personal and interpersonal aspect. This more personal dimension is made more explicit by other tutors:

> "(experiential learning is)...Putting someone in a situation that they may not have been in before so that they can experience what it feels like."

> "It is that form of learning in which students take an active part, learning from their own experience."

> "(experiential learning is)... a means of gaining an awareness of what may be happening or maybe gaining certain values from an experience which is purposeful, such as what it is that you might be doing with another individual, such as an interactive process."

These tutors appear to be alluding to the idea that experiential learning may be a more **personal** form of learning than may be the case with other sorts of learning. Sometimes this comparison and

85

contrast with more "traditional" forms of learning was made more explicit :

> "I see experiential learning as having less cognitive input, less cognitive assessment and more input from the people who are involved."

> "I think that there are differences between more traditional ways of doing things and experiential learning. With experiential learning, there is something that can happen and you make use of it. And for me it is more like doing therapy than teaching, because it allows me to utilize what they (the students) bring as people into the situation and you can't pre-plan that."

Here we see the accent on personal experience and on modifying teaching and learning methods according the emerging needs of the students. Again, such an approach to learning and teaching may be traced to the humanistic school of psychology and to the "Romantic" school of curriculum planning (Lawton 1973). Lawton contrasts the Romantic school of curriculum planners with the Classical school. The Romantic school was characterised by the advocacy of student-centred learning.

The student centred approach emphasises negotiation with learners of learning objectives and evaluation techniques and also negotiation of learning and teaching methods. In this school, **learning** is seen to be the key issue (as opposed to **teaching** being the key issue in the Classical school. The writers that are associated with the Romantic school often blur the distinction between learning and therapy. Carl Rogers, for example writes of both concepts in each of his books on the psychotherapeutic process (Rogers 1952, 1967, 1983). John Heron also makes no distinction between the two concepts, arguing, instead, that all psychotherapy is a form of learning and thus learning techniques can embrace psychotherapeutic techniques (Heron 1989a). The nurse educator cited above seems also to be blurring the distinction when he suggests that :

> "...for me it is more like doing therapy than teaching, because it allows me to utilize what they (the students) bring as people into the situation and you can't pre-plan that."

Two assumptions appear to be being made here. First that teaching is rather like doing therapy and that you can't pre-plan what happens in learning (and, by implication, in therapy). This style of carrying out therapy, of not pre-planning the aims or outcomes of therapy is very much in line with the humanistic approach to psychotherapy (Rowan 1986, Perls 1973). These humanistic therapists, borrowing from the existential concepts discussed above, work from the premise that people are dynamic and ever changing. Thus, given the difficulty of pinning down human experience in any way, the focus of therapy shifts from session to session. The respondent, above, appears to be applying such a process to learning and to nurse education.

All of this can be contrasted with Lawton's (1973) Classical school of curriculum planning. In the Classical school, the locus of power in planning and executing a curriculum (aims, methods and evaluation procedures) remains with the teacher. The reason behind this is an epistemological one. The Classical curriculum developers (and Lawton cites Peters [1972] and Hirst [1972] as prime examples) would argue that knowledge is external to the one who does the knowing. That is to say that knowledge is "objective": it "exists" independently of the knower. Thus, by way of trivial example, the simple mathematical truth that, under normal circumstances 2+2 = 4, remains true, regardless of the person who knows it to be true. For the Classical curriculum planner, then, education is concerned to a large degree with the passing on of a whole range of "truths". This can be done in a relatively impersonal way. The educator, here, is one who helps to induce learners into "ways of knowing" (Peters 1972). Education is concerned with this passing on of ways of knowing and is never compared in the literature with therapy. It would appear that the Classical tutors make a clear distinction between education and therapy in ways that Romantic tutors do not.

The Classical approach, then, is a totally different approach to the Romantic one. As we noted above, the Romantic approach, borrowing as it does from existentialism and phenomenology, tends to encourage a point of view that knowledge is "relative" and that what we know is inextricably bound up with **who we are** and how we view things. Now, whilst this does not seem to be very apparently the case if we consider the 2+2 = 4 argument, above, it may become more apparent when we turn to the domain of feelings, perceptions, beliefs and values. It may be possible to argue that **both** types of education have their place : that the classical approach is appropriate

87

for the passing on of "factual" information and the Romantic approach is appropriate for what Heron (1983) calls the "education of the affect", for here, too, we see a divergence of thinking between Classical and Romantic tutors.

Classical education is more concerned with the domain of knowledge, whilst Romantic education is often concerned with exploring and "educating" the emotional aspects of the person. That some of the nurse tutors were concerned with this domain of affective education is illustrated by the following quotations :

"For me, as I said before, it is, it has been documented as an effective way of attaining affective objectives..."

"In a nutshell, I would say it is more of a focus on the emotional side of the individual and their personality."

Arguably, this focus on the emotional aspects of the person would be an anathema to the Classical curriculum planners who would see emotional involvement as a potential hazard in that it would tend to mitigate against rationality. The Romantic curriculum planners would, on the other hand, be particularly interested in helping people to explore emotions as part of the educational process, arguing that any attempt to split the person into a "cognitive" element and an "emotional" element is necessarily false.

In summary, it may be noted that a number of the respondents had difficulty in defining the term "experiential learning" and a number defined it tautologically. Those who **could** define it tended to talk in terms of :learning in the here-and-now, learning from past or present experience, learning through direct, practical experience or in terms of it's involving "personal learning" of some sort.

Experiential Learning Methods

If the nurse tutors sometimes found it difficult to **define** experiential learning, they had less difficulty in citing examples of what they would call "experiential learning methods".

Examples of experiential learning methods could be divided into two groups :1) experiential learning in the clinical setting and 2) those activities which nurse tutors use in schools of nursing. The respondents talked more of the second category than of the first.

In the "clinical setting" category, some respondents talked of how they worked in the clinical setting, alongside the students as a means of encouraging and teaching them :

"...We work with them on the wards quite a lot and you can see then whether they have picked up what you would have expected them to have picked up and learned what you would have expected them to have learned in experiential learning situations."

This respondent appears to be alluding to a set of learning objectives or criteria for learning that she has in relation to the student nurse and that one of the purposes of working with learners on the ward is to ascertain the degree to which they have or have not met those objectives or satisfied those criteria. Whether or not those objectives or criteria where made explicit and discussed with the learners was not pursued by the respondent.

Another respondent continued the theme of working in the clinical setting as being an example of an experiential learning method:

"another experiential learning method is when the students work on the ward and actually taking the temperature of a patient".

In this example, no mention is made of whether or not the educator sees it as part of her role to work in the clinical setting with the nurses in question. Another educator made explicit the distinction between experiential learning methods as working in the clinical setting and experiential learning methods as methods that are used in the school of nursing:

"I see experiential learning methods as means of helping people to learn through experience and either within the work situation or within a more formal situation - in the classroom."

Here, the classroom setting is perceived as "more formal", presumably in contrast to the more informal learning that takes place in the clinical setting. The reference could also be an allusion to the tutor's own perceptions of the differences between classroom and clinical learning. Another respondent also made a distinction between the formal and the informal modes:

"In the wards and taking temperatures. That would be an example of an experiential learning method. (To the interviewer:) Or do you mean in a formal learning context?"

The bridge between **particular** types of experiential learning methods used in the school of nursing (such as role-play) and "clinical" types of experiential learning methods was made via experiential learning methods that **simulated** clinical settings. One educator described such practices graphically:

"If you want a nurse to know what it feels like to be a patient, you stick them on a ward and stick them in bed and let them experience that."

What may be noted, here, is a certain **tone** of response. The educator uses the word "stick" to describe the process of helping a nurse to experience the process of being a patient. This use of language in this way is thrown into relief by another respondent who suggested that:

"My feeling is that you must not forget the fact that those people sat in front of you are people who are experiencing something : not just your voice but their environment, relationships with those around them, how hard the seat is, how hot the room is..."

It is always difficult to determine the degree to which what people say reflects attitudes and beliefs but it is interesting to ponder on the degree to which the use of language in this way is indicative of particular attitudes towards students, learning and education.

The "bridging" method of experiential learning, through simulation is also described by another respondent:

"We do some practicals. We, for example, get some of them to act as patients and nurses. And the patients we give various problems to, like telling them they are blind or telling them they are paralysed down one side. And

the other students who are "being nurses" have to feed
them and then we talk about what it felt like to actually
by fed when you aren't capable of doing this yourself
and how the people acting as nurses treat people who
are acting as patients."

Here, various elements of Kolb's (1984) experiential learning
cycle may be noted in practice. First, the respondent sets up a
simulated clinical experience and asks students to adopt roles. Then
they act out a particular experience. Afterwards all the "actors"
gather together to reflect on the process and draw out new learning
from that reflection.
A more dramatic form of simulation of patient
experience was mentioned, in passing, by another respondent, as:
"Getting nurses to spend one night in a hospital bed".

Such simulations of patient experience are well documented in
the literature on nurse educational practices (Langford 1990, Dowd
1983, Schafer and Morgan 1980). All of these references, however,
refer to **descriptive** papers that offer a "how to do it" approach to
setting up and evaluation simulations of this sort. There appears to
be no published studies, to date, that empirically evaluate this method
of teaching nurses.

Experiential Learning Methods Used in the School of Nursing

Whilst, as we have seen, a number of the respondents described
experiential learning methods as those that involved learning in the
clinical setting, others used the term to described teaching and
learning methods that they used in the school or college of nursing.
Sometimes, the definition of experiential learning methods was very
broad and all encompassing :

"Experiential   learning   methods   are   things   like
simulation, role play, games, project work, seminar -
they are all experiential forms of learning as opposed to
where the learning is just a receiver of information".

Here, the respondent appears to be making a distinction
between "information giving" as a form of teaching and "something

91

else", which is not so clear, though the suggestion is that a distinction is being made between "information giving methods" and "activities based" methods. All of the methods that the respondent cites as examples of experiential learning methods involve the learners in some sort of activity (simulation, role play, games, project work and seminar), although it might be argued that the seminar is less of an action technique that the other four.

This accent on activity is developed by another respondent who appears to grappling with the concept of using personal experience in education:

> "Experiential learning methods involve actively participating in something which may involve actual physical activity. Another method would be bringing your own experience, what you have learned from an experience you have had - perhaps into a discussion group from which other people might be able to learn, so everybody is bringing their own experiences...so perhaps a discussion group would be a form of experiential learning as well....I think that anything were one takes an active part in it rather than sitting back and being told...(is an example of an experiential learning method)."

What is also notable about this extract is that the respondent appears to be clarifying her thoughts as she speaks. She appears to be discovering examples of experiential learning methods as she talks through the topic. This is evidenced by her saying '...so perhaps a discussion group would be a form of experiential learning as well. This possible uncertainty over what are and what are not examples of experiential learning methods (or, looked at a different way, this "thinking on your feet" approach) was evident in other respondents :

> "...a seminar in the school...I think that's probably an experiential learning method, would you say?"

> "Project work is an experiential approach, I think...I don't know if everyone would agree with that..."

> "...on the other hand, a demonstration or something in which you take part is experiential, isn't it?"

A number of things may be happening here. It is possible that those people being interviewed were uncertain about what constituted an experiential learning method. It is also possible that they did not carry around in our heads examples of particular methods (although all the respondents knew that the researcher was going to interview them at a particular time and all knew that the topic was "experiential learning".) Another possibility, as we noted above, is that, during the course of an interview, the respondents discovered or thought more clearly about what an experiential learning method was and what it was not. Yet still it is possible that the term "experiential learning" has been defined so liberally and widely in the literature that the term can be used to cover almost any activity. It is worth recalling Knowles (1980) listing of experiential techniques, cited in a previous chapter of this book :

> group discussions, cases, critical incidents, simulations, role-play, skill practice exercises, field project, action projects, laboratory methods, consultative supervision (coaching), demonstrations, seminars, work conferences, counselling, group therapy and community development. (Knowles 1980 : 50)

One other possible explanation for some of the respondents' hesitancy may also be explained by the fact of their knowing who the researcher was and of his interest in the field. In this sense, it is possible that they may have been trying to offer "right answers" or seeking reassurance that they were on the right lines in their responses. Short of the researcher adopting some sort of disguise or employing an anonymous research assistant there seems to be little that can be done to combat such a problem (if it is, indeed, a problem), short of the researcher assuring respondents that he is seeking **their** views and perceptions : an assurance that was offered to each respondent in the present study.

Role play was frequently cited as an example of an experiential learning method:

> "Other examples would be setting up a role play where either the persona adopts a different role or their own role and examines how they felt or what happened as a result of that role play."

This respondent distinguishes between two sorts of role-plays: the sort in which the player is asked to adopt a different role from his current one and the sort in which that player remains "who he is". A similar distinction is sometimes made in the literature between role play and psychodrama (Goble 1990). Typically, in role play, participants are asked to imagine themselves in roles other than their own, whilst in psychodrama, participants act out situations that they have lived through or which they are likely to live through. These varieties of "role play" are referred to by another respondent :

"The experiential learning method I use most, I guess, is role paly. If we are dealing with a specific situation like teaching a group of students basic nursing skills, for example, what I would be doing with that group of students would be enabling them to set up a pseudo situation, a generalisation of a clinical situation in a classroom when **they** took on, either the roles of the nurse or the roles of the patient."

Another respondent talked of the "invention" aspect of role play - of the setting up of a contrived situation in order to enhance learning through experience:

"The methods I have seen have been mainly role-play. The role-play techniques that I have used were always ones that were constructed. They were sort of directive, I suppose, they were structured. I became aware, through my involvement with a psychodrama therapist of the use of socio-drama and then my techniques became more or less unstructured - unstructured in the sense of non-directive, because I think that we were able to construct situation that had be experienced by people in the group. And we were able to put them into an action format through drama."

This respondent appears to be making the distinction between role play and psychodrama (or "sociodrama"), alluded to above. She also appears to be suggesting that psychodrama, or encouraging group members to "play themselves" and to draw on their own experiences is beneficial and requires less structure and less direction from the facilitator than does role play. Another possibility is that this respondent became more secure or comfortable in using the approach and consequently became less structuring and directing.

Other methods, apart from and sometimes along with, role play were cited as examples of experiential learning methods :

"Things like role play, structured exercises, group work, people working in pairs or threes, exploring concepts and students bringing their own experience to bear in relation to the concept that is being looked at."

"The methods I have used from the very beginning have been exercises, albeit ones of relaxation, meditation, trust type and icebreaking activities as a means of enhancing people's relationships with one another."

These respondents refer to activities and exercises that involve the students in interaction with each other - an approach that has received much attention in the literature on experiential learning (see, for example, Heron 1982, Knowles 1981, Boydel 1974). These respondents and the others cited above also place emphasis on the need to include learner's own experience in the learning situation. It would appear that the activities described here (role play, structured exercises and so on, have become part of the normal repertoire of educational techniques for some nurse tutors to the degree to which one respondent could describe one experiential learning activity that she used as :

"the old cliche thing like "blind walk"..."

The "blind walk" activity is one that involves learners being blindfolded and lead about in order to experience what it is like to be blind or to explore senses other than the visual one. It has been widely described in the literature (Kilty 1982, Burnard 1990, Heron 1982). Another respondent referred to the activity as one of a variety of role-play situations :

"We get some of the students to act as patients and nurses. And the patients we give various problems to, like telling them they're blind or telling then they're paralysed down one side..."

95

Not all of the respondents refer to these "traditional" experiential learning methods. Some appeared to extend the term "experiential learning methods" to include many other approaches. For example, one respondent said this:

> "If you send them (the students) to the library to get the answer to a question, and they are interacting with each other around books off the shelves, I would call that an experiential learning method."

This respondent describes what appears to be a fairly traditional teaching method of encouraging students to gather information for themselves but identifies the **interactive** aspect of it as the "experiential learning" part of it. Indeed, the one issue that seems to be common to almost all of the respondents identification of experiential learning methods is the accent on **interaction**. This factor has clear links to the literature on experiential learning which has tended to emphasis the use of such methods for enhancing interpersonal and communication skills (Kilty 1983, Heron 1982, Burnard 1990, Marshfield 1985.)

Sometimes more traditional teaching methods were cited as examples of experiential learning methods:

> "The experience of doing a project, doing the work, is an experience in an educational setting...project work is an experiential approach, I think."

> "It depends how far you want to describe experiential learning methods, I suppose. I mean, you could say that if you listen to a lecture there are experiences you could pick up."

> "(when talking about experiential learning methods)...There is also the Open University packs as well, distance learning packages..."

Here, the notion of experiential learning methods has been extended to include project work, lecturing and distance learning, though it is notable that such expansion was the exception rather than the rule. As noted above, when asked for examples of experiential learning methods, most respondents talked of role play, structured group activities and other similar interactive activities.

Finally, in this section, it is interesting to note **negative** definitions. In other words, to note what the nurse tutors suggested **were not** experiential learning methods. The most frequently cited example of what was **not** an experiential learning method, was lecturing :

> "Traditionally, I guess, the non-experiential methods of learning would be where the teacher stood on front of the class-room, students traditionally behind desks."

> "I would say a lecture is certainly not an experiential learning method."

The other factor that seems to have emerged, however, (an this is alluded to in the first quote cited immediately above), is the issue of teacher-centredness and teacher control. A number of the tutors referred to the lecture method and the more traditional approach to teaching and learning being concerned with the teacher being in control of the learning situation and deciding what does and what does not go into the learning encounter. Indeed, it is interesting to note the use of the word "teacher" in these extracts and to note that the descriptor is rarely used in other contexts throughout the interviews. Given that the term "teacher" is possibly more frequently associated with schools and with the teaching of children (whilst the words "tutor", "lecturer" and "facilitator" are more often used in the context of adult learning), it is possible that some of the respondents associate lecturing and teacher-centred learning with the education of children. This would be in line with Knowles" writing on 'andragogy" or the theory and practice of the education of adults (as opposed to "pedagogy" or the theory and practice of the education or children) (Knowles 1978). Notable features in the following quotes are the locus of power, the issue of relationships between teacher and students (and vice versa) and the question of passivity versus activity on the part of the learners.

> "I see non-experiential learning as one in which there is minimal or no student involvement in the direction in which the teacher goes. So, if you like, it is non-student-centred"

"(examples of non-experiential learning methods would be) teacher-centred approaches, teaching, lecture, seminars..."

"Tutorials are less experiential because primarily they are geared towards clarified cognitive contents in relation to the cognitive/intellectual objectives".

Whilst the phrase "geared towards clarified cognitive contents in relation to the cognitive/intellectual objectives" is far from clear, the above quotes are indicative of what the tutors counted as "non-experiential". It is here that we may perceive a "boundary" in the process of definition, for whilst it is clear that role play, games and simulations fit clearly into the "experiential learning " camp and lectures fit clearly into the "non-experiential learning" camp, the **seminar** is mentioned both as an example of an experiential learning method and as an example of what is **not** an experiential learning method. If we consider those characteristics that the nurse tutors feel that activities such as role-play and games have in common and what it is that characterises the lecture (and acknowledge that the seminar sits on the boundary between those two groups), we may be nearer to identifying what sorts of things nurse tutors are describing when they discuss experiential learning methods.

It would seem that those methods described by the tutors as experiential learning methods are characterised by activity, interaction both between tutor and student and between student and student, and an emphasis on personal experience as a starting and finishing point of the educational encounter. On the other hand, the lecture seems to be characterised as a method that allows the tutor to decide on content, allows him to control the lesson and has a tendency to encourage only one-way transmission of information : from the teacher to the student. The seminar (typically, in which a student adopts, temporarily the role of the teacher-as -lecturer, whilst the teacher remains in overall charge of the learning group), seems to have some of the characteristics of both types of learning encounter.

These, then, are ways in which the nurse tutors **defined** experiential learning and experiential learning methods. In the next section it will be useful to explore the tutors **theories** about the experiential approach.

Theories About Experiential Learning

The nurse tutors offered a wide range of theories about experiential learning as they talked. In this section, the following categories emerged : general theories about learning, theories about experiential learning, theories about the nature of personal experience, theories about student choice in learning, therapy and experiential learning, emotions and experiential learning and, finally, theories about self-awareness. In this section, each of these categories is discussed in turn.

General Theories About Learning

One common theme about learning was that not everybody learns in the same way. Thus, one respondent suggested that :

> "Well, I don't necessarily think that everybody learns in
> the same way or at the same speed or for the same
> reason..."

Thus suggesting a multiplicity of motives for learning and ways of learning. Another said that :

> "I don't think you can say 'yes all the class have learned
> to do that. All the class may have been taught how to
> do that...I think people have different learning speeds
> and methods of learning. Some people learn better by
> reading from a book. Some people learning better by
> doing."

This respondent seems to be making a clear distinction between **teaching** a topic and someone having **learned** as a result. In one sense, the two can be separated in this way. The activities of teaching, on the one hand, can be separated from the activity of learning, on the other. Peters (1972), however, argues that it is not logical to have said that you have **taught** something, unless learning has taken place as a result. In this conceptualisation, learning is a necessary part of teaching.

Another respondent took a similar view of alternative ways of learning when he stated that :

"I think you've got to provide many different ways of learning the same thing. So that if someone learns better by reading it out of a book, they'd better read it out of a book, as well as, you know, having an experience."

None of the respondents **developed** this theme of individualised learning and it has to be reported that the researcher did not attempt to "draw out" those respondents further. It is open to conjecture to what degree such beliefs about the multiplicity of learning styles and learning methods was based on rational theory or on research based knowledge about the learning process and to what degree it could be classified as "armchair philosophising" about educational processes. Also, if a number of the respondents felt that people learn in a variety of ways, it would be interesting to find out the degree to which they modify their own teaching and learning methods in response to that variety.

Theories about Experiential Learning

In this section, various theories had been put forward about such things as how experiential learning approaches should be used, how it should be managed and how it should be evaluated.

Some respondents felt that a structured approach to learning should be adopted by the person who used the experiential approach :

"I always give them specific tasks to do, observation tasks. Although I have found that what happens is that the better the role play, the less they remember what their task was."

Here, the suggestion seems to be that although structure is imposed by the teacher, as the students develop their roles, they get "lost" in the role play and get drawn into it to such a degree that they loose the sense of structure that they started with. However, for the above respondent, the need to return to structure is important :

"...you end up doing 20 minutes of, say it is a real difficult one (role play) like one we did recently with general students. After about 20 minutes we asked them for observations. The majority had forgotten all about that because they had got so involved in what was going on...That was OK, that wasn't a problem, because in fact we would have been able to instruct them to do what they did."

On the other hand, the respondent then seems to relent on the issue of structure and to suggest that involvement is more important. He continues :

"You can't give instructions to **become involved.** That naturally had been generated by the intensity of the role play. That was probably more useful at the end of the day because we had really gripped them and we were able to talk about that - a live issue, even though it was a role play."

It could be argued, however, that the respondent still retains overall control over the structure by suggesting that "we" had really gripped them : it was not the role play itself that had cause the total involvement, but the way it had been set up by the teachers.

Another respondent talked of the need for structure but seemed less clear about what the structure was for or even what the **aim** of the session was. For him, the setting up of a role play itself seemed all that was necessary :

"We just set the situations up and put the students in them and hope that they will learn something and give us some feedback. And we try to tell them what we expect them to have learned. Whether they actually did or not - I think that's very individual."

The respondent seems to have an aim in mind when he suggests that he tells the learners what they should learn but then the whole process seems to become rather vague : "whether they actually did or not - I think that's very individual'. Again, too, there is reference to the general learning theory discussed briefly above, that people learn in all sorts of different ways. This tension between aims and outcomes and the uncertainty of the process, is echoed by another respondent who suggested that :

"You hope that the experience that you give them will give them the learning that you want them to achieve - (if you can understand that) and I don't think that that is necessarily always right"

The respondent goes on to explain how experiential learning methods, in giving people different experiences lead to different outcomes.

What **may** be happening here is a tension between the teacher as the organiser and bringer of structure to the learning situation and the teacher as facilitator or one who stands back and lets things happen. This conflict is described well by another respondent, thus :

"Learners might see you as **the** teacher. The teacher has certain authority because, through the social role, there are certain role behaviours which are prescribed for tutors. And there are certain things that you must fulfil. Experiential learning de-emphasises that. We know it is there but we don't make it as though it is the most important thing there. I think first and foremost what experiential learning does is to help us see each other as people first, rather than as a person in a particular role with a certain authority over me or somebody else."

This respondent then went on to discuss the idea of **lessening** structure rather than maintaining it and seemed less concerned about the issue of **what** was learned or what the learning outcomes were. For him, one of the aims of experiential learning appeared to be the meeting of persons and the stripping away of role expectations. "Personal sharing" and self disclosure were issues that were discussed by a number of respondents :

"I don't thing you can kind of go in there when you are doing experiential learning and expect not to share yourself, to some extent..."

"I think it is important that groups that you work with, you are able to retain your image or how people perceive you as a teacher but at the same time to get close enough to them to want them to involve themselves in that kind of thing and I think some

102

teachers find that difficult because they have a
perception of themselves in their teacher role and then
they find getting close to students...I suspect that it is
more difficult for people who have been a tutor for a
long time."

In the last response, we see the coming together of a number
of issues discussed above. The respondent discusses something of the
change of role that is required (whilst maintaining that it is possible
to "retain your image..as a teacher". He also talks of the need to get
closer to the students and to get to know them better, whilst
suggesting that this may be difficult for those who have been tutors
for a long time.

Considering these issues, it seemed that many of the
respondents were felt that experiential learning was concerned with
a changing structure to the learning situation, a change of role for the
teacher and with a close relationship between learner and teacher.
This **personalised** form of learning is discussed by many educational
theorists from the "Romantic" school of thought (as discussed in the
earlier part of this chapter). Certainly, as we have already noted,
Rogers (1983) tended to talk of "facilitators of learning" rather than
of teachers and Heron (1983) of the "education of the affect". For
both of these writers, the idea of the teacher having a close and
personal relationship with his or her students is an important one, as
is the de-structuring of the traditional role of the teacher. One
respondent took this personalised approach to learning to the extreme
when he argued thus :

"It wouldn't be difficult, really, unless we come to
semantics, to separate the term 'experiential' from
"existence". That is the way I see it. People don't seem
to think of it, but to me it is very obvious, life itself is
experiential. You have to experience life to meet life.
Whether you are actively participating or not, you are
experiencing life. So to **live** is to experience it. This is
the way I see it."

Here we notice something **very** personal going on. Two
"personal" things are noticeable here. First, the respondent says,
twice, that "this is the way I see it" and then he notes that "People
don"t seem to think of it...but to me it is very obvious.." It would

seem that **this** person has adopted a particularly personal view of the experiential learning process. Also, too, the respondent has broadened out the concept of experiential learning to take in the whole of life experience. "Experiential learning" has become synonymous with life itself. Also, the respondent is using language in a fairly idiosyncratic way : "So to live is to experience it". This issues of the use of a particular sort of language is discussed in a later chapter under the heading of Learning the Language.

Another "personal" view of the approach was taken by another respondent but in a rather different way. In his discussion of the nature of experiential learning, he noted, unprompted, that :

> "I don't think there is much (experiential learning) going
> on in other parts of the country. I may be wrong but it
> is based on the feeling that I often get requests from
> other places to come and talk to them about it because
> they don't understand it. The only other place that I
> think something may be going on is Y..."

This was an interesting response given that the respondents were spread through different counties of England and Wales and given that the survey discussed in the following chapters of this book suggest that **many** people have used or taken part in experiential learning approaches. This response could be a one-off response from someone who does not take account of the "larger picture" of nurse education. On the other hand, it could also be part of the process of **personalisation** that seems to be linked to the experiential learning process. Just as the previous respondent was able to report that (in his view) "People do not seem to think of it in that way...", so this respondent felt that "I don"t think there is much going on in other parts of the country" and...."they don't understand it". This leads us on to the theories about personal experience that emerged out of the interviews. What ever experiential learning is **not**, it **does** seem to be very markedly to do with personal experience.

Theories About the Nature of Personal Experience

A number of respondents indicated that they felt that **personal experience** was an important aspect of experiential learning. That is to say that they suggested that a student should experience something for his or herself rather than only being **told** about something :

> "I don't think that people can understand it to the depth in which they need to just by being told about it (counselling, nursing). I think there has to be some putting the feet into the water. Even in a role-play situation, that is more likely to enable meaningful insight to occur in the student than if I just tell them something."

This respondent was able to elaborate on this notion of personal experiencing as distinct from only receiving theory :

> "If I talk to them about theory, just theory, and make it quite dry, I think they are less likely to learn from that than if I give them clinical experiences. Just me telling them there are steps along the way... they are unable to integrate for themselves. But I do think that process of integration is more likely with the increased involvement of experiential learning."

The "increased involvement", for this respondent, appears to be the factor of the student being personally involved in the learning encounter. This involvement in the learning process is stated slightly differently by another respondent :

> "If you take basic learners, the majority of their time as a student is experiential learning because they are not in a class, they are on the wards. Nevertheless, it is recognised in nurse education that the learner - by being a nurse- so it is actually the hands on practice..."

This respondent seems to be suggesting that experiential learning is something to do with "hands on practice", of work in the clinical situation as an example of how to learn nursing. Another aspect of personal involvement as **arising out of** experiential learning, is described by another respondent :

> "I think it would be better if they actually felt it because...you think you can imagine what it would feel

like to role play something but I think until you actually
do role paly it... most of the students get caught up in
the role they are playing and experience feelings that
they may not have realised that they would do."

There are echoes, here, of the quality referred to in the
previous section, that of becoming "caught up" in what is happening
and becoming "lost" in the role play or activity. What seems to be
emerging is a suggested difference between traditional "learning of
facts and theories" and "learning, personally, through direct
involvement". This "personal learning" is discussed in some detail in
the literature. Carl Rogers (1983), for example, describes his concept
of "experiential knowledge" or knowledge that is qualitatively
different to the memorisation of knowledge handed on by a teacher.
Given the discussion by a number of the respondents about this
different "quality" of learning, this "personal learning", it is probably
not suprising that many felt that students should exercise a degree of
choice about whether or not to become involved in an experiential
learning situation.

Theories About Student Choice

As we have noted, a number of respondents referred to the personal
nature of the learning that takes place under the heading of
experiential learning and often described the idiosyncratic and
individual nature of students' responses in such learning encounters.
This lead on to discussions about student choice in experiential
learning. The issue was tackled from a number of points of view :

"Obviously people make a personal choice about how
much to divulge of their experience...I think it is really
important to actually give them an opportunity, give
them some space and permission to share the effects
that the experiential learning has had on them."

Here, the issue is that students should be given the opportunity to talk
about what happens to them in an experiential learning encounter,
although the decision about **what** they disclose should be left to the
individual student. A number of respondents were explicit that no

student should be coerced into taking part in experiential learning sessions :

> "The facilitator will have a responsibility to let them know that they don't have to (take part). The students need to have that confidence to be able to decide. But if they weren't told in the first place, they wouldn't want to come out with it first and say 'Really, I don't want to do this" because their notion of teaching-learning relationships was still that kind that they had at school."

There are echoes, here, of the earlier issue (discussed above) of changing roles in experiential learning and of students bringing to a new type of learning encounter an "old" model of the relationship between student and tutor. Also, though, is the point that teachers (or "facilitators" for this respondent) has a duty to ensure that students take part in experiential learning activities freely and of their own choosing. In order for this to happen, the student must know that such an option exists in the first place. This insistence on voluntariness is discussed by a number of commentators. Heron (1982) proposes the use of a "voluntary clause" at the beginning of any experiential learning session. He suggests that it is always made explicit that no student will at any time be forced to take part in an experiential learning activity and that at all times participation is voluntary.

However, one respondent noted that offering this voluntariness may take courage on the part of the inexperienced tutor :

> "Funny, I have been waiting to see, or expecting, most of the individuals in a group to say "I'd rather not do that" and then it would be impossible to do the exercise. But it hasn't happened yet. And yet it would be my fear and that could be a danger to the facilitator who is not very comfortable yet in using experiential methods. He may not actually tell learners that they have the right (not to participate) because of the fear that most would abstain from participating."

The fear of students not taking part in experiential learning activities seemed to prove groundless for that respondent. His own experience was that people did take part when offered the opportunity

not to do so. Another respondent found this aspect of choice and important one and one that had implications for other aspects of the students' lives :

> "It can be very liberating, in the sense of people being made more aware of the options in their lives. They can possibly make choices more systematically, once they see that they **can** make choices."

The fact of being offered a choice at all, seems to be an important one for that respondent and the suggestion is that one such choice can lead on to others, although why such choices should become more "systematic" is not clear. Traditional learning methods in nurse training have not normally included an "opting out" clause or voluntary clause. More usually, students are expected to take part in lessons and lectures and the argument is sometimes used that students should take part in learning encounters because a) they are undertaking a formal training and b) they are being paid for their attendance. This is in contrast to colleges of higher education and universities where the accent on compulsory attendance and participation is not the tradition.

The issue for the respondents, here, is not just whether or not students should **attend** experiential learning sessions but that, given the personal nature of experiential learning, students should not be forced to **disclose** their thoughts and feelings to others and should be able to reserve the right to decide when and if such disclosure takes place. One respondent appears to be suggesting a gradual approach to such disclosure :

> "You could have them to it privately, to begin with - write it down - and they would share it with somebody else in the group. You could, as it were, extend the concept of experiential learning into that process of de-briefing and evaluation. Then there could be group discussion if you want to."

In his interview, this respondent discussed the importance of students being allowed to take their time over self-disclosure and that the process of self-disclosure should not be rushed - a point made by Jourard (1964) in his length discussion on the nature of self-disclosure. Whilst self-disclosure is important as an educational activity for

108

Jourard, he is also adamant that no one should be encouraged to self-disclose too quickly. It is possible to imagine, however, that such self-disclosure is self-limiting. Presumably few people will make self-disclosures against their will. On the other hand, perhaps some people get caught up in the "disclosing atmosphere" and disclose too easily and too much (Cox 1978).

Therapy and Experiential Learning

One respondent expressed concern over whether or not experiential learning sessions could become psychotherapy sessions. This is a point that develops directly out of the issue of self-disclosure, for self-disclosure is necessarily an important element of almost all of the psychotherapies (Sherffen 1978). The respondent raised a number of issues on this matter :

> "I think when you start turning things into therapeutic situations or where the teacher sets themselves up as a "guru", as a fount of wisdom...I think that's taking education too far. Unless everyone is agreed that that is what everyone wants to do and everyone has gone there with that in mind...The worry is that in most situations in nurse education, people have no choice - even though they may appear to be offered it..."

Here we see an anxiety about the teacher-as-facilitator misusing his or her role and becoming a "guru" figure (presumably with considerable charismatic power developing through that role). When this guru relationship develops, according to this respondent, the issue of choice becomes a little more blurred. R.S. Peters (1966) discussed just this point after suggesting that the teacher who became a guru figure no longer produced critical thinkers but "followers" who were more likely to accept the guru-teacher's ideas than question them. Whilst the guru relationship is more commonly associated with religious sects and cults (Milne, Burdett and Beckett 1986), it is interesting to note that Wallis (1984) classifies the Human Potential Movement as one of the "new religions". The Human Potential Movement is a portmanteau label that covers many of the strands of thinking and action in humanistic psychology. It was noted in the first chapter that much of the theory and practice of approaches to

109

experiential learning derive from humanistic psychology. This respondents anxiety about the development of gurus may be a reasonable one. Many writers on education in the humanistic field also discuss therapy in the same volume (Rogers 1983, Maslow 1972, Heron 1982). Heron has also suggested that therapy is a form of education (Heron 1977b) and although whilst he does not reverse the equation, he suggests that he does not find it useful to make a distinction between the two. The two, related, issues of gurus and therapy seem to be ones that are addressed somewhat obliquely in the literature.

The respondent, above, also seems to be suggesting that the guru relationship and the question of therapy are acceptable if everyone in the learning group are agreed that that is the relationship expected and the purpose for meeting. A contractual issue arises here. It may be argued that groups of students meet together for the purpose of learning nursing and not for the purpose of therapy. If they are unwittingly offered therapy, then, arguably, the person who offers it is going beyond the contract that he or she has with that group of students. Much will depend, of course, on whether or not that person and that group of students would want, like Heron, to subsume the notion of "therapy" within the larger notion of "learning". The idea of "therapy" is not addressed as an issue in any of the National Boards' syllabuses of training nor is an issue that arises in books on curriculum development in nurse education.

Emotions and Experiential Learning

The question of whether or not experiential learning should or should not shade over into therapy is complicated further by the fact that many of the respondents discussed the **emotional** element of experiential learning. Given the personal nature of some elements of experiential learning and given that students are sometimes encouraged to self-disclose their personal thoughts and feelings, it is perhaps unsuprising that emotions sometimes come to the surface. Indeed, much of the literature on the "humanistic" approach to experiential learning discusses, explicitly, the advantages of emotional release as part of the experiential learning experience (Heron 1973, 1982; Rowan 1988). The respondents in this study seems to have some ambivalence about the issue of whether it was or was not appropriate for students to express strong emotions in a learning situation :

"It hasn't happened often (crying). On one occasion it happened and it was quite difficult. One thing that I wanted to do was to stop it spreading...that we'd all end up tackling this particular problem. There was a danger that we'd all become involved in the drama that was going on in this person's life. I think what I did was to play it down at the time and then saw her afterwards and had a chat about it."

Here, the fear seems to be exactly that the learning session was liable to become a therapy session : "there was this danger that we'd all become involved in the drama that was going on in this person's life". Therapeutic groups actively encourage such involvement (Whittaker 1987). Another respondent reported :

"I know one of my colleagues has jumped in and touched raw nerves in certain people and has not been able to handle that...these sorts of things tend to occur sometimes. But the group themselves have been alienated from that person (the colleague).. So I tend to stick with a safe one because I don't feel at the present time that I am skilled, if that is the word to use, into entering into any more deeply...into the areas that touch on the emotions."

This respondent seems to be noting that his colleague was not particularly popular for stirring up the student's emotion, he notes his own lack of skill in handling these sorts of situations but also seems to be questioning the **appropriateness** of working in the emotional domain, by his querying whether or not "skill" is the appropriate word to describe the handling of emotional situations.

Another respondent talked about what he perceived as the dangers of an over-emotional learning environment :

"If a person has a very good relationship with his personal tutor, then he can just come back and see them whenever he wants but if you haven't got that relationship, then they might tend to go off with all their feelings ploughed up about something and not feel there is anyone to talk to afterwards."

Another hinted at emotional aspects of experiential learning but seemed to move away from the area thus :

"That is not to say that there isn't an emotional element in them. It is just that there hasn't been any over-emotional outcome."

What is difficult to judge, here, is who is defining the issue of "over-emotional". As it is a teacher speaking, then presumably, it is that teacher who is deciding that an outcome is or is not "over-emotional". What remains hidden is how the students perceive the issue of the emotions in experiential learning. This question of the difficulty of judging levels of emotional arousal was addressed by another respondent who said:

"It is difficult to judge, of course, whether or not an issue is threatening. For example, if you just ask 'What makes you feel bad?' or "What have you felt sad about recently?", there is always the danger that you may get into something that is very unpleasant."

Another also illustrated the "unknown" potential for emotional distress in experiential learning :

"This group of general learners had been given all sorts of specific observational tasks to do but in fact they all ended up crying and it all got quite difficult."

The issue of emotional release in experiential learning sessions seemed, overall, to be focused on two things :

- whether or not emotional release was appropriate in a learning environment and should or should not be encouraged,
- whether or not a nurse teacher had the necessary skills to handle emotional release if and when it occurred.

Self-Awareness

In the literature, much reference is made to the use of experiential learning approaches as the means of developing self-awareness (Heron

112

1982, Kilty 1983, Burnard 1985, Kagan, Kay and Evans 1986). In this section, it was noted that various respondents identified the use of experiential learning methods as the means of students identifying their own needs and wants and developing self-awareness as a result. The concept of self-awareness is problematic. Questions need to be asked about what is meant by "self" (Williams 1973). Then, if the notion of "self" is problematic, questions need to be asked about what it is that one becomes aware of when one becomes self-aware. In the 1982 Psychiatric Nursing syllabus (ENB 1982) these issues were not addressed. It seemed to be assumed in that syllabus that the notion of self-awareness was not only unproblematic but also that it would be readily understood by readers of that syllabus.

The first extract illustrates a dialogue between the researcher and a respondent on the issue of what self-awareness is. The respondent, prior to this excerpt, had suggested that experiential learning methods were useful for enhancing student's self-awareness:

Researcher So what is self-awareness?

Respondent Awareness of one's own needs, one's own wants, one's own fantasies. Awareness of what affects other people, awareness of others as well is tied up with it. What other people's needs and wants are and so on. I keep talking about wants and needs and I am thinking now that they are both feelings - there is a feeling side to that. And feedback, I suppose, are the main things, and being in contact with reality and not being in a world of your own...

Researcher What does that mean?

Respondent What, reality?

Researcher Staying in contact with reality.

Respondent With me, it means being in touch with the effect of oneself on others and observing in others how you affect them. And seeing wether there is any correlation between that and between the individual's. I think somebody who is totally unaware of how they affect others is a little bit out of contact with reality and to some extent isolated and alone and possibly in need of help.

This respondent is able to articulate a view of self-awareness as being one that involves awareness of one's own view of one's self and also an appreciation of how others see one. He was also suggesting that the "person who is in touch with reality" is also a person who takes account of **other people's** needs and wants. This altruistic view is echoed by another respondent, who used the expression "personal development" to describe part of what he was trying to achieve through the use of experiential learning methods :

Researcher : So what is personal development?

Respondent : Personal development, the way I see it, is the process whereby an individual grows in self-awareness and ability to relate empathically to others. I am pretty concerned about the definitions of empathy. I don't see empathy as being total. I see it as being a balance of being able to be with another person and yet to be quite separate, with the recognition that you can never fully understand another person...Some definitions of empathy seem to me to be almost a compulsive helping. "I have got to be with the other all the time". That would seem to deny the reality of being with oneself, self-concern, self-awareness, assertiveness. I seem to be going round in circles here..."

This respondent seemed to be struggling with concepts of self-development/ self-awareness and the need to demonstrate empathy. On the other hand, he is acknowledging what he claims to be the impossibility of complete empathy. Empathy had been identified by Rogers (1967) as a necessary and sufficient quality of a therapeutic relationship, whilst Kalisch (1971) suggested ways that empathy could be developed in student nurses. On the other hand, Mackay and Carvar (1990) in an extensive review of the literature and research on empathy could find no agreement as to how empathy should or could be accurately defined. Rather like the concept of "self", in self-awareness, it seems that the concept of "empathy" could be a slippery one.

114

Another respondent took much more of an individualistic approach to the question of experiential learning and self-awareness. He suggested that in considering the experiential learning approach :

> "I recommended it not so much for the skills but for what it has done for me. It has actually integrated and synbooked a lot of loose ends, put me more in touch with my weaknesses and how I can go forward in my own life...which is not an easy thing to do when I want to do my own thing but at the same time I want to accommodate you. It is quite difficult."

During this interview, it was sometimes difficult to know whether or not the respondent was using experiential learning methods for his own or his students development, and this tension is reflected in this extract. The respondent uses language in a particular way to describe concepts that are not easily pinned down in terms of their meaning : "It has actually integrated and synbooked a lot of loose ends..." Exactly what the respondent means here is impossible to assess without further questioning. Use of language in this way is discussed in a later chapter of this book, where the researcher develops a theory of particular language styles in some approaches to experiential learning.

Using Experiential Learning

Rationale for Using Experiential Learning Approaches

In this section, respondents identifies general explanations of why they use an experiential learning approach. First, a fairly broad and general explanation :

> "[I use them] partly because they were done here before I came by the other staff. Partly because I can remember learning things when I was training to be a nurse that I learned how to do because we did them and had fun while we were mucking about, making beds with people. But also because they are something I've never

115

forgotten, therefore I think that's why they are a good learning exercise."

This respondent appeared to be reflecting on his rationale as he developed it. He works from a position of "because they were used before..", to the fact that they are fun, through to his remembering things from his own past that he never forgot. In a sense, the respondent is identifying many of the stages of the experiential learning cycle identified in the literature : learning from past experience (Kilty 1983), reflecting on past experience (Kolb 1984, Kilty 1983) and developing new theory out of past and present experience (Kolb 1984).

Another respondent developed the rationale of using experiential learning methods because he enjoyed using them. He suggested that he used them because :

"I enjoy it. I think that is my main reason, although I am well aware that you can't just do things because you enjoy it. It must be beneficial as well. But I...have got the very naive belief that if I am enjoying the way I am teaching, I am much more likely to be effective. I think there is a point at which that isn't true, like if I am leaving people behind, or if I am just doing things or saying things because I find them interesting or amusing..."

The respondent takes a less "naive" view than he would let us suppose. Indeed, for him to acknowledge that he is "naive" in this way, is to raise a certain irony : if he **were** naive, presumably he would be unaware of it, by definition of the term. What he goes on to suggest is that he cannot simply use experiential approaches just because he enjoys them, but also that he accepts responsibility for ensuring that his students "stay with him". Another respondent echoed this "fun" element :

"I feel happy with them. I feel confident in using them. I find them fun and I find them very useful to learn and as far as I am concerned, learning is fun."

Another respondent noted that his rationale for using them changed as he became more experienced :

116

"I used to use them for the sake of using them - 'try this because it is something new' - but I must admit that in the last year or two I don't use them so often now.   I tend to try and work things on a workshop basis...a thematic thing and if there is room for an activity...I look for ways of presenting parts of it experientially."

This respondent, during the course of the interview described how he had changed from a "total" experiential learning approach to one that incorporated elements of both more traditional **and** experiential approaches, rather in the way that Butterworth (1984) had recommended.   Another respondent acknowledge that he used experiential learning approaches but :

"...not a lot. If I am teaching science subjects, perhaps anatomy and physiology, its difficult to role play that...but then I would use things like setting syndicate work for them, where they actually have a certain set task...whether you would call that experiential learning, I don't know."

Here, having said that he didn't' use experiential learning approaches very much, the respondent went on to ponder as to whether other learning methods could be described as "experiential learning" - again pointing up the difficulty of defining experiential learning. The question of **how much** teaching and learning is experiential, was developed by another respondent :

Interviewer   Would you say, then, that experiential learning methods can be used right across the board for all topics, for some topics or for very few topics? How would you place them on that sort of continuum?

Respondent : About 50%, I would think...it would need a bit of ingenuity on the part of the teachers and facilitators to do any more than that. Some subjects just don't lend themselves to experiential learning.

This leads on to the question of what topics and subjects experiential learning methods **were** used for by the respondents.

Using Experiential Learning Methods

In the previous section, the debate was more about the question of using experiential learning methods at all. In this section , the focus is more on **the ways** in which such methods were used. Sometimes, respondents used them for particular topics :

"I think it teaches management techniques."

"I use them for things like counselling - counselling skills."

Some respondents doubted the applicability of experiential learning approaches to certain topics, particularly to the teaching and learning of anatomy and physiology :

"I think if you look at pure sessions such as anatomy and physiology, I think you would find it more difficult to drag in always the ideas of the experiential learning concept."

"More of the general things like bacteriology, biology, anatomy, physiology, dietetics and straightforward psychology - these are best done by other methods..."

It is interesting to note the first respondents' description of anatomy and physiology as "pure" and to note the seconds' expression "general things like" - it is almost as if both were comparing those topics with other sorts of topics (perhaps with the "softer" topics of interpersonal skills and communication studies) but this must remain speculation as no further explanation was offered or sought. Meanwhile, another respondent took a very different view :

"I think experiential learning is applicable to every subject. All the topics - even biology - are taught experientially."

This respondent is suggesting that experiential learning is applicable to **all** subjects and also underlines that it is applicable to biology. It is as if the respondent might be in some doubt that it could be applicable for this topic. On one occasion, the approach seemed to be used for personal reasons :

> "At the top of my list I would put experiential learning activity. Experiential learning is probably my prime interest."

Like the previous respondent, this one had no hesitation in recommending the widespread use of experiential learning methods for all topics.

Another respondent took a different approach to the issue of what to use experiential learning methods for. She suggested that, rather than tie them to particular topics, choosing them was dependent upon whether or not they were appropriate as a learning or teaching strategy :

> "It's like any sort of teaching or learning, isn't it. You have to decide what you want them to get out of it and then the best way to achieve that end. And if its experiential learning, you work it out that way."

This respondent's approach not only differs in its implication that you don't have to tie methods to topics in teaching and learning but also implies more control by the teacher. It will be recalled that much of the literature on experiential learning is concerned with negotiated learning and with allowing students to puzzle things out for themselves (Brookfield 1986, 1987, Boydell 1976, Rogers 1983). This respondent took a more structured approach in suggesting that it was the teacher who decided what the students were to learn and who then decided on the appropriate method. An anxiety about whether or not experiential learning approaches allowed you to maintain control in this way was voiced by another respondent :

> "When you're teaching students, I suppose you have to be open and trust them to do what you want. You can stop at an appropriate time and draw out the experience or draw out what they should have learned. That's another thing. If they haven't actually achieved what you expect them to, you've got to salvage something from the situation, haven't you?"

119

This issue of the 'teaching in control of the learning environment' was echoed by a number of respondents :

"You have to stop them now and then and get them to explain how they feel and you have to wind them down again or debrief them afterwards.'

"You need to give them a sort of strategy and allow them to feel successful."

"You have to let people know where they are going and what's expected of them."

"If problems have occurred its because the session hasn't been properly structured. People haven't known what the boundaries are."

This issue of structuring, boundary maintenance and organisational control by the teacher was clearly an important issue for a number of respondents and in some contrast to the tendency, in the literature, towards allowing the students to structure their own learning and learning approach (see, particularly Rogers 1983 and Kilty 1983).

Students' Responses to Experiential Learning

Predictably, perhaps, not all students responded to the use of experiential learning approaches in the same sorts of ways. One respondent reflected on the range of responses thus :

"There are all kinds of reactions. I would say that there are some that are very resistant to that approach and don't want to know. You get the whole range. You get, I would say, the majority are interested in it. If you wanted a percentage on it, I would say perhaps 75% enjoy it and another group, perhaps 15-20% are cool towards it and dubious and wonder whether it is of any value to them."

Others noted a positive response to the use of experiential learning activities :

"Well, they have a good time. They have a giggle and a bit of fun."

"Some group, if you gave them the choice, they would spend the whole block doing experiential stuff."

Some, however, noted more negative responses and for a variety of reasons. One felt that experiential learning methods did not suit everyone and this was the cause of some students feeling uncomfortable using them.   Note, however, the word that this respondent uses to describe the students :

"I think the other thing is that acting and experiential learning doesn't suit the audience sometimes..."

Consciously or otherwise, this respondent identified a class of students in terms of an "audience". This metaphor and the notion of acting, is taken into account by another respondent who acknowledge that an air of artificiality was sometimes noted by the students :

"It's not like the real thing', is the classic statement."

It will be noted in the following chapter which identifies the perceptions of the students, that this often **was** the classic response. Other respondents noted this credibility problem :

"I think some of the other difficulties they have is that they can't see the immediate connection between doing role play and the usefulness of that in their work situation."

"[Some of the problems are] being on display, not understanding the connection..."

The allusion to acting and the stage was developed by another respondent :

"Some people are just shy, they just don't like getting up in front of six people, let alone nineteen others, and play

121

acting...They don't like that. They don't like being up on the stage, as it were. "

Sometimes, problems associated with the use of experiential learning approaches were put down to the students' familiarity or unfamiliarity with them. If they were used from "day one" in a course, then they were more likely to be positively responded to by students :

"I was of the opinion that if you started with people from the beginning, that they would be fully receptive to it and they would take it on board and they would be pleased as anything with it. But this is not always true. I think it is the way it is introduced and if you help people to understand the value of it."

"Sometimes they respond with some apprehension, if they haven't used them before. And because of this, we usually start with something that is quite humorous, ice breakers and games with no other purpose than to get them used to experiential methods of learning. And then, when we get on to the more serious things, they become **very** cooperative : they like it."

"I think what it depends on is how they were first introduced to it."

There were hints, though, that experiential learning methods had or could be misused, although no respondent was particularly keen to elaborate on just how. With one respondent, it seemed that he had known of colleagues who had used very dramatic, emotionally demanding activities that forced the students to confront some of their fears and which were a compulsory part of the curriculum. The "black arts" side of experiential learning in terms of forced catharsis and of people being encouraged to self-disclose as much as possible are discussed in the literature (Liberman et al 1973, Masson 1990, Cox 1978). Those researchers and authors claim that such involuntary participation in emotional and pseudo-therapeutic activities can be psychologically damaging. They also question the ethics of leaders of such groups forcing their particular set of values and beliefs on group members. This respondent, though, was loath to elaborate too much and this raises interesting questions about how far a research should continue to probe a respondent. In the current study, the researcher took the decision that it was best **not** to probe on what was sensitive issue for the respondent. The hint of problems in the past came via the following exchange :

> **Interviewer** How do students generally react to experiential learning activities?
>
> **Respondent** I don't have any problems (laughs)
>
> **Interviewer** : You laughed just now. What was that about?
>
> **Respondent** : I was thinking about the people...I have said to people 'We will do something experiential now'. People tend to groan because they have had bad experiences in the past.

Another alluded to a hospital that he had worked in where he considered that experiential learning had also been misused, with the result that :

> "I remember one particular class who absolutely hated role play. The minute they heard the words "role play" they said "Oh no. Not again." And they just didn't want to participate."

Again, the respondent was loath to discuss the issue further but in this later case, it sounds as though role play may have been overused as a teaching and learning technique to the extend that the students disliked it.

Sometimes, reactions to experiential learning were seen in terms of the students' previous socialisation into learning and teaching methods. This appeared to work both positively and negatively :

> "Sometimes you get the 18 year olds who are much happier with it because they have done that type of stuff at school and it is nothing new for them."

"I guess some people, within their previous formalised teaching such as when they are in school or college before they come into nursing, are more used to a formalised setup, where they have notepads and you provide them with diagrams..."

One respondent linked her own uncertainty with the methods with the reception she got from the students :

"Because I wasn't terribly relaxed within myself, I think it was transferred to the learners and they were just as tense as I was. Although they would go through with it, maximum learning didn't take place."

This respondents last comment leads into the next category of response : that of evaluating experiential learning.

One particularly idiosyncratic response to students responses can be reported, although it is difficult to comment on it. It may be that the respondent is using language in a particularly "personal" way; that he is describing problems from a particular theoretical standpoint unknown to the researcher or that he is engaging in the use of language in terms of "Learning the Language" discussed in a later chapter. It is included here for completeness :

"I have got all sorts of very strange responses that, because you get similar effects as you do in trance-induction and time-distortion effects : place-distortion effects and I have used that as a technique, for actually, before I talk about the theory of something, to get them to experience as similar state, without the necessity of me doing anything with them."

Evaluation

Evaluating learning has been an important feature in the educational literature (Clift and Imrie 1981, Hamilton 1986, Patton 1982). There are a variety of issues within the concept of evaluation. The term can cover, at least, the following issues :

● effectiveness of teaching,

- whether or not students valued the teaching session,
- whether or not learning took place.
- the effectiveness of a course.

Item 1) above refers more to the technique of teaching, whereas, item 3) refers to whether or not students learned as a result of the teaching that took place. Peters (1966) argues that it is a contradiction in terms to say that "teaching occurred, but no learning took place". For Peters, at least, to teach is to ensure that people learn.

At the outset, it is important to discriminate between evaluation and assessment, although at times the two are used synonymously. To evaluate is to place a value on something and in the educational context, it is usual to talk of evaluating teaching or courses. Assessment, on the other hand, usually refers to identifying the progress (or lack of it) that students have made in the educational process. Thus, by way of shorthand, it can be said that tutors evaluate courses and assess students (Rowntree 1988)

The most frequently referred to concept used by the tutors in this study and in this context, was that of "feedback". The term has origins in the field of electronics but has come to be associated with a group of students disclosing how they feel about an aspect of learning to each other, or to their teacher (Rowntree 1977). By far the most frequent approach to eliciting this feedback was to ask the students at the end of an experiential learning session what they thought of it :

> "At the end of the session, whatever it is that we happen to be doing, I either have a structured feedback mechanism whereby you ask each individual for comments about what he experienced."

> "Feedback, essentially : you listen to what they learned from it, at the end of the session."

> "At the end, we draw out what the good points and the bad points were and how they felt about these experiences and hopefully make it meaningful to them so that they will remember them and so that they can use the experience."

This aspect of inviting people to reflect on what has happened to them and then to verbalise those reflections, echoes Kolb's (1984) and Pfeiffer and Goodsteins' (1982) approaches to experiential learning, as discussed in the first chapter. An essential feature of those authors' experiential learning cycles was the "reflection and publishing" stage.

However, as may be noted in the last extract above, many tutors were uncertain about the effectiveness of their evaluation procedures. Sometimes, this was stated in passing, with the suggestion that **no** evaluation procedures were particularly effective :

> **Researcher** : What about evaluation?   How do you evaluate the experiential learning?
>
> **Respondent** : Not very well. I think it is evaluated in the same way that other sessions are evaluated, by verbal feedback and written comments...

Sometimes, though, the doubts were developed by the respondents. One, for example, doubted whether it was possible to evaluate learning sessions directly after they had taken place :

> "I always make sure that we have a de-briefing period, a sharing period or whatever, at the end. What you evaluate there is people's immediate response, not the long-term response and you are not evaluating the finish of the process. I think it is easier to evaluate non-experiential learning..."

Another noted the subjective nature of the whole process:

> "It is a bit difficult because it is, of course, subjective - how people feel...At the end of a fortnight, you have got the time to cogitate and reflect, and they write down their feelings, both individually and collectively. But it is, we realise, a subjective business."

Others reported that they found the question of evaluation a difficult one for a number of reasons. These reasons, though, were not always clearly explicated :

"Evaluation is a difficult thing. The nature of it is not easy. Experiential learning is about experience. It is about life and therefore it has to be an individual thing."

This respondent seems to be referring to the subjective, personal nature of experiential learning but seems to get caught up in the difficult of expressing what he found difficult. For others, the question of evaluation was one that should be reflected back to the students, thus continuing the tradition of student-centred learning (Rogers 1983) :

"I can't see why the students or the people concerned can't ask themselves how they want to evaluate it. How are we going to know that this has been useful today?"

Another, reported a hearing of a similar view, although finding that he disagreed with it :

"I was told by someone that experiential learning shouldn't be evaluated – that the coming together of the experience, the make sense of the experience should be something going on in the individual without any interference from other people or formalised in any way. However, I disagree with that person."

The respondent went on to describe his evaluation process as involving feedback at the end of the session, as with the respondents reported above. This style of having "evaluation rounds" at the end of experiential learning sessions is widely reported in the literature (Kilty 1983, Burnard 1985, Heron 1982, Dietrich 1978). The usual format for such as process is follows : each person in the learning group is encouraged to say what they liked **least** about the session. This is carried out in the form of a "round" whereby each person speaks in turn. This round is then followed by a second in which each person, in turn, states what they liked **least** about the session (Dietrich 1978). This may be followed by a general discussion of the session or by the closing of the session.

Sometimes, the evaluation process included the tutor or lecturer joining in the process. The following respondent used the descriptor "we" to describe his and his students' involvement in the process :

"At the end of each exercise, we go around and we evaluate what we felt we have learned or what effect an exercise had on us...we share that. At the end of the learning period we then evaluate **each other** and we evaluate ourselves..."

This process seems to incorporate both self-disclosure on the part of the students and tutor or lecturer and feedback from other people. Luft (1967) has suggested that the necessary conditions for developing self awareness are those two elements : self-disclosure and feedback from others. He argues that once we describe our personal feelings to others, and once we hear other people's evaluation of us, we are more likely to develop a balanced view of who we are. In the case cited above, the respondent seems to be going beyond evaluating the experiential learning session and introducing the notion of self and peer evaluation (Heron 1982, Kilty 1983).

Of all the comments on evaluation, however, the clearest message that came from the respondents was that evaluation of experiential learning was difficult :

"Yes. Its a very difficult thing."

"The evaluation of experiential learning is very difficult"

"I think it is a problem...you tend to evaluate it in the longer term...incredibly difficult to do...how on earth can you evaluate?"

Advantages of the Experiential Learning Approach

One of the most pervasive aspects that was to come out of the interviews with the tutors in this study was their **enthusiasm** for experiential learning. Often, they chose the experiential learning approach because either they enjoyed it, or they appreciated the increased involvement it allowed them with students :

"The person orientation - I love it. I like being involved, I like the students as people..."

"The advantages, the main advantage, that you can guarantee that everybody is active, it is active learning - which you cannot guarantee when you are just standing in front of a class."

"I think it can be fun. I think it can be exciting. I think people **like** doing it. Usually, I find that people love it."

Another advantage that was often cited (and in sharp contrast to what the **students** had to say on the matter) was that of "realness". Many tutors felt that experiential learning had a "real" quality that was missing from more traditional methods of teaching and learning:

" I think the advantages are that it's as **real** as you can get. Sometimes it is real. It's actual, real experience. There is no transfer problem with that : it's real. It happened or it is happening."

"Yes, it's real. If it's **not** real, it's as near real as you can get it. Therefore people can try things out, perhaps develop skills and try skills out in a safe situation."

The "realness" referred to here seems to be in contrast to the lack of realness in more formal learning approaches. Alfred North Whitehead (1922) wrote of "dead knowledge" and of how teachers were very good at passing on such dead knowledge. He suggested that, in fact, "knowledge keeps no better than fish." The respondents, here, seemed to be suggesting that what made experiential learning real, was the fact that students were bringing to the learning situation their own thoughts, feelings and experiences rather than rote learning "dead knowledge". However, one respondent was not quite so enthusiastic on this point and expressed the view that :

" I am sometimes a little sceptical of whether people actually give you the truth when you ask them what their appreciations of their experiences or their understandings of what we have been trying to do."

The respondent is raising an issue that seems to have been neglected in the literature on experiential learning approaches to education. Most of that literature refers to the sharing of experiences

129

by participants, but most tend to take it on trust that people will tell the truth about those experiences. Rogers (1983) seems to take a particularly optimistic view on this issue when he suggests that what needs to happen is for the teacher to **trust** the students and then they will be more self-disclosing. Jourard (1964) took another optimistic view when he suggested that "self-disclosure begets self-disclosure". However, what remains unquestioned is that when people do self-disclose, they will necessarily be honest. Sometimes this perhaps rather naive view percolated through the interviews :

> " I am very open with the students. I don't pretend to be able to do any more than they do."

> "The advantage as far as I am personally concerned is that you can share things together ; yourself with the learners, learners with yourself..."

> "It leaves everybody free, relaxed with each other, more honest with each other."

Whilst the idea of a comfortable atmosphere and a relaxed approach seems likely to promote self disclosure in group therapy settings (Whitaker 1987), it does not necessarily follow that when people disclose in the fairly public setting of an educational group, they will **automatically** "be more honest with each other". One respondent illustrated a seeming lack of honesty with his students when he reported that :

> " It also provides responsibility for one's own learning, so it de-emphasises the fact that it is the teacher's responsibility for them to learn and **without having to say so,** I found learners just take it on board, without having to be taught. I have to get whatever is possible out of it and yet **you don't have to tell them that.**"[emphases added]

The respondent seems to be suggesting that the responsibility of the teacher is reduced in experiential learning and yet it is not necessary to openly declare the shift in responsibility and the change of emphasis in learning. It was noted in identifying the **disadvantages** of the approach, that confusion sometimes occurred because students and others were not always sure about tutors motives and aims. These disadvantages will now be discussed.

Disadvantages

The tutors identified a number of disadvantages of the experiential learning approach and these were fairly diverse in nature. Some felt that **appropriateness** was sometimes a problem :

> "Yes, people might abuse it in the sense that they may use inappropriate methods in terms of it is not appropriate for the group they are working with and it doesn't necessarily meet the needs of the group, whilst it may be meeting the needs of the teacher." [emphasis added]

This response echoes the problem highlighted in the last paragraph of the last section : it was possible to ask who preferred experiential learning methods the most, the students or the tutors? Sometimes the appropriateness issue was seen in terms of experiential learning being a bandwagon or a passing fashion :

> "Some see it is the be all and end all in education. It is a panacea in terms of you can teach anything with experiential learning. I am not convinced about that. And some people may abuse it. They may use certain methods or approaches which may be inappropriate to the group."

> "Everyone is jumping on the bandwagon - a whole concept which is being taken on board and people using what is dangerous stuff sometimes."

The "dangerous stuff" was sometimes made more explicit :

> "Some people can't cope with doing anything like role play in front of other people. Some people clearly do have unpleasant experiences. You never **quite** know what you are tapping into when you set up an

131

experiential exercises...You never **quite** know what you
are going to unlock."

"I am not awfully happy with T groups and encounter
groups etc. Apart from any other reasons, people don't
have the skills to defuse the situation afterwards. So I
am not too happy with those."

The last respondent, above, referred to T and encounter groups
that represent fairly dramatic forms of group experience. Although
the use of the term "encounter group" has been used in a variety of
ways (Smith 1980) it is usually traced back to the 'T' or training
groups of the social psychologist Kurt Lewin (Shaffer 1978). Lewin's
T groups were not therapy groups but were designed, instead, to help
managers and executives within large organisations to become more
sensitive to the interpersonal and group-dynamics aspects of their
work (Lewin 1952). There were, however, similarities between T
groups and therapy groups, for the T group member was introduces to
group dynamics, not through didactic instruction but by personal
participation in the group experience.

This format of running intense, emotional small groups of this
sort became popular with a wider clientele and developed in the mid
1960's at the Esalen Institute in California and at the Center for
Studies of the Person at La Jolla, California (Kirschenbaum 1979). At
the La Jolla centre, Carl Rogers further developed his own style of
client-centred counselling in a group format and called it a **basic
encounter group** (Rogers 1970).

Whilst Rogers was developing this basic encounter format,
William Schutz, at the Esalen Institute was developing what he called
open encounter (Schutz 1967, 1971, 1973). What characterised Shutz's
groups was that they allowed for almost total expression of feelings
and thoughts, positive and negative and relied heavily on the
expression of strong emotion (or catharsis).

The effectiveness and value of the encounter group is far from
clear. Postuma and Postuma (1973) compared samples attending
encounter groups, structured classes in human relations and no training
at all. Ratings made after training and again six months later showed
no differences between the groups in rate of negatively evaluated
changes. Back's (1972) study of encounter movement saw the function
of the encounter experience as largely cathartic. He was unimpressed
by the findings of evaluation studies concerning long-term effects of

groups, but considered that short-term group experiences proved so compelling during the "boom" encounter years of the late sixties and early seventies because such encounter groups offered precisely what was lacking in many people's everyday lives : excitement, intimacy, and a clear sense of purpose.

The point, here, is that many of the experiential learning activities described in the literature can be traced directly back to the encounter group movement (see, for example, the activities and exercises offered by Heron 1982, Kilty 1983, Burnard 1985, Kagan, Evans and Kay 1986). As noted above, many of the respondents worried about "things getting out of control" or of not being sure "what your going to unlock" or of "encounter and T groups". The unifying factor, here, is that many of the activities that grew out of the encounter movement dependent upon catharsis, or the free expression of emotion. Many of the respondents in this study felt unsuitably prepared for the role of handling such emotional release, if it occurred. Or, as one respondent suggested :

> " I suppose that one disadvantage is that you would trigger off something and the facilitator might not recognise it and the person goes away without being given an opportunity to talk about it and understand it and not being given any aftercare."

Sometimes, respondent's worried about whether or not students might feel pressurised to take part in certain activities :

> "In a sense, there are many pressure on them to take part that as soon as I say ' I don't want to take part in this exercise - it's too threatening'...it takes guts to say that and I think that as soon as you've said that, everyone's going to wonder 'well, what's wrong?"

Overall, the issue of uncertainty about emotional expression or things getting out of control was one of the most frequently discussed disadvantages of the experiential approach :

> "There's a danger that your students might get upset"

> "To force a group of people to expose themselves - I personally couldn't do that. I dare say it has it's uses,

133

but it's not something I'd be happy about. I feel quite strongly about that."

Learning to Use Experiential Learning Methods

We noted above, that a number of respondents expressed doubt as to whether or not they could handle some of the situations that might arise out of using experiential learning methods. This leads to the issue of how tutors came to be prepared to use such methods in nurse education. Often, the training was minimal or they learned by using the approach themselves :

> "I don't know if you can actually train. I find that most of what I use now, I learned from other tutors and working with them and seeing how they do it and how they cope with it and trying it myself."

> "...the role has no formal training as such"

> "Just by trial and error, unfortunately. I say unfortunately because we have all experienced negative and positive things. It can have disastrous results, although it depends on what topic you choose and whether you think you are skilled or not. You are your own monitor as far as that is concerned.

For these respondents, the whole issue of training was a rather "hit and miss" affair, although it could be said that they learned to use experiential learning methods experientially - by direct, personal experience. Not many of those who learned in this way felt themselves to be adequately prepared, which raises a nice paradox about the notion of learning from personal experience. One the one hand, it seemed to be an important value that students were encouraged to learn from direct experience, often in an informal, unstructured environment. On the other, many of the tutors felt that **formal** training in experiential learning methods would have helped them.

" I would have loved to have gone on an experiential
learning methods course, which I think would have been
very much to my advantage."

Sometimes respondents had come across experiential learning
methods during their tutor's courses at teacher training colleges,
although the amount of time allocated to experiential learning on
these courses seemed to be variable, as did the outcome and the
reception :

"While I was at (name of college), I spent one full day
so-called "being taught" how to use experiential
methods. That was a laugh really, it really was. We
knew better methods than what they were trying to
impart to us."

"I suppose (my training) would add up to something like
120 hours, I suppose. Some of it was new, some of it
was old stuff that I knew myself anyway."

" When I was on the tutor's course, (name of teacher)
used to take us for relationship skills and I got quite
involved in that. I didn't particularly enjoy it that much
at the time. In some ways I found it a bit difficult and
a bit stressful."

It is interesting to note that the tutors often expressed
dissatisfaction in their training in experiential learning methods or
that they had "done it before" and yet all were committed to using
experiential learning methods with their students. One respondent was
very positive about the training he had received in a variety of
experiential learning techniques and used the "evangelical" tone that
can be identified in much of the humanistic literature on experiential
learning and which will be returned to as a point of discussion in a
later chapter :

"It was like reincarnation. I found the (name of teacher)
approach very confronting...confronting techniques that
I could drown in...Co-Counselling to me is the best
method...the power is with the client...Recently I have

been learning in other areas, other doings : regression, how to actually manage regression..."

This respondent was undertaking a lengthy diploma course in experiential learning methods and was quite clearly "sold" on the concept of experiential learning in nurse education. What made his interview difficult was that he frequently used the "language" of the humanistic approach to experiential learning, which has to be understood in order to make sense of what the person is talking about. As we have indicated, this issue is taken up in more detail in a later chapter.

Influences

In this final section, it was noted that the tutors sometimes referred to authors that had influenced them in their use of experiential learning methods, although the research quickly found that asking questions in this area was not necessarily productive :

> **Researcher** : If you turned to the literature, what...'
>
> **Respondent** : Like a test! Can you remember the title? We have got a big pile of books in our office that we did into and I wouldn't actually claim that I have used any of those to a great extent that it would be worthwhile saying : 'This is a book I have used'.

When influences **were** mentioned, the following writers were cited and are presented in rank order : Carl Rogers, John Heron, Pfeiffer and Jones, Philip Burnard, William Schutz, Gerard Egan and John Stevens. Regarding the last two authors, Gerard Egan has written books about counselling and helping relationships (Egan 1990) and John Stevens wrote a book of exercises and activities based on Gestalt therapy methods (Stevens 1971). The other writers have been discussed or cited in this book and could broadly be described as belonging to the humanistic approach to experiential learning.

Conclusion

In summary, it can be said that although some of the nurse tutors found experiential learning difficult to define, many of them felt that it was an active and personal form of learning. They felt that it involved emotional responses and encouraged self-awareness. Generally it was viewed as an enjoyable form of learning but it could sometimes be unreal and embarrasing. Finally, it usually involved **facilitation** rather than teaching.

7 Students' perceptions of experiential learning: Part two

This chapter describes the findings from the secondary analysis of the students' interviews, using the method described in chapter three.

The Students' Perceptions

The student nurses' interviews tended to be shorter than those carried out with the nurse tutors. The students were generally less immediately talkative than was the case with the tutors. Also, they talked about experiential learning in different ways. Early on in the analysis of the two sets of data it became apparent that it would not be possible to use the same sets of categories for the two groups. Instead, the following list of categories emerged from the students' transcripts :
1. Definitions of Experiential Learning,
2. Learning in the Clinical Setting,
3. Experiential Learning in the School or College of Nursing
4. Role Play
5. Other Experiential Learning Methods
6. Advantages of Experiential Learning and Articulating What Experiential Learning Is.

Definitions of Experiential Learning

Some students seemed to echo what they thought their tutors thought experiential learning was but then were able to make their own modifications of those definitions :

> "Well, here in the school, the way the tutors seem to see it is say you had a session and it would be like practical things - sort of trying - through the experience you got - trying to make you learn something relevant to whatever, but I suppose in the broader sense, like, you know, working on the wards and things like that."

> "By the practical experience we have in school and I always think of it as what I learn on the ward and talking to the qualified staff about it. Discussing it with them."

Such definitions made the researcher, at the analysis stage, wonder about the degree to which the students had been "primed" to any degree about the issue of experiential learning. It is possible to imagine that the students had received prior notice of the researcher's visit and had wanted to know what he was going to ask questions about. It is also possible that the question was then raised by some students as to what experiential learning was. One respondent appeared to have done more homework than most on this issue when he said that :

> "Only a few days ago, I was asked did I wish to come and see you - I just went and got your book out and had a look up under "experiential learning" to find out what exactly what you had written about it because I had always thought experiential learning was basically just learning from doing rather than learning by having it told or just programmed into you."

Following this interview, the researcher decided to ask some of the respondents what they felt that researcher's motives to be in asking questions about experiential learning. This lead to a fairly broad set of possible reasons being mooted :

"Your intention, I should imagine you are trying to get to find out what I really feel about, rather than just having me to reel off various key words and expressions which I have picked up from books. You want me to be more honest."

"I feel that you are doing it for your research project and I feel reasonably safe doing it. It's got nothing to do with this hospital, anyway."

"I suppose that you're trying to find out which methods are better - whether people learn more in school or in the wards."

The notion of experiential learning as something more than "just being taught" was identified by other respondents. Also (and this mitigates against the suggestion made above, that the students were "primed" in some way) nearly all of the students had very different perceptions of experiential learning when compared to the tutors. What makes this important is that it will be recalled that the students were drawn from schools of nursing in which those tutors worked. Other definitions of the "more than teaching" sort, were as follows :

"It means learning which differs from sort of conventional classroom instruction, in that it is something which you use when you use your own experience and you learn from what you've done in the past or you actually learn by going through a practical procedure or some exercise. So it is learning which is centred more around yourself and your life than sort of text book stuff."

"Well it's different from the old style of teaching, rather than the emphasis being on the individual to develop the way they should develop or the way they want to develop, the emphasis in traditional teaching is on a person standing in front of them and giving their views."

By far the most common form of definition, however, was the type that identified experiential learning in terms of learning in the clinical setting, or sometimes as a combination of "school" learning and "clinical" learning :

"By the practical exercises we have in school and I always think of it as what I learn on the wards and talking to the qualified staff about it. Discussing it with them."

"Well, simply learning by experience. I would have thought of it as over in the school doing role play and I would imagine it would be on the wards left to your own devices as far as the tutors are concerned."

In the above two extracts, we see the hint of two issues that became important ones in the study : a) the student's view of the clinical situation and the clinical staff and b) the student's view of the tutorial staff in the school or college of nursing. Many researchers have noted the importance of the clinical setting as vital in the process of learning about nursing (Orton 1981, Ogier 1982, Fretwell 1982 Gott 1984,) and this study confirmed, to a large degree, the centrality of both the clinical staff and the clinical setting in the learning process. The clinical emphasis was to be found in other respondents' responses :

"Experiential learning involves a wide environment of skill [sic], particularly on the wards."

"Well, practically anything that's actually practical and involves doing things is experiential learning, in my opinion - any type of nursing that I've actually done or come across on the ward has been experiential learning to me. What I don't regard as it, is learning from books and things - anything theoretical, I don't classify **that** as experiential learning".

Notable in the last extract, is the differentiation between learning on the ward and "theoretical" learning. Experiential learning, for this respondent, was associated with "practical" things.

On the other hand, sometimes a more individualistic approach was taken to defining the field : personal learning and the process of learning from life experience, as suggested by some of the nurse tutors:

"Well, I think experiential learning includes absolutely everything. I think you could argue that your entire life is a learning experience, you could classify anything as experiential learning. Were you thinking of something specific?"

This respondent's question of the research is interesting as it suggests that the game of 'guess what's in my head' was going on between respondent and researcher (Holt 1964). Holt argues that it can be frequently noticed that students try to anticipate the "right answer" for the teacher by "reading the signs" or checking for clues as to what that teacher might want as an answer. In this interview, it seemed possible that the respondent was trying to please the researcher by coming up with the "correct" answer.

The individualistic, "personal" approach to experiential learning was taken by another respondent who suggested that :

"I suppose my views of experiential learning are actually trial and error, by yourself with nobody else telling me what or what not to do."

This was reminiscent of some of the tutor's descriptions and of the humanistic approach to experiential learning which had emphasised freedom of choice and the primacy of personal experience (Rogers 1983, Rowan 1988). On the other hand, one student saw the whole issue of experiential learning as one of passing fashion :

" I haven't really got a real definition. If you like, it was just a word, a concept which was just thrown around a lot, you know, almost a trendy thing to be used in the school. I just think of it in those terms."

Although the respondent went on to say much more about the process of experiential learning, it is interesting to note this scepticism - perhaps suggesting that the concept of experiential learning had been discussed with him and his colleagues by an enthusiastic tutor. This observation of the "trendiness" of experiential learning was noted by another respondent :

> "It's quite popular at the moment. Quite the 'in thing',
> I suppose."

Reflecting back, for a moment, it was interesting to note that one of the tutors had **denied** experiential learning's "trendy" image, thus :

> "I think it is going to go on. I don't think it is going to
> go away. It is not a 'fashionable' thing. It has made a
> steady increase since the sixties and will go on growing."

This tutor (from a different school of nursing to the above students) was more certain about the permanence of experiential learning than were the students. Also notable was this tutor's reference to the roots of the experiential learning approach in the 1960's.

The themes of learning from personal experience - particularly in the clinical settings were developed further by all the respondents and it is to that issue that the discussion now turns.

Learning in the Clinical Setting

It quickly became clear that the students felt that they learned most about nursing from working in the clinical setting. This was often of more importance to them than were the activities carried out in the school of nursing. One student summed this up most completely when she suggested that :

> "Well, I suppose that's the job you have got to do and
> obviously the people on the ward are actually doing it.
> And you are sort of there, aren't you?"

This student invokes a rather passive view of the learning process. For her, it seemed, the process of "being there" was enough in itself. Others developed this theme :

> "I mean, on the wards you learn by...you don't learn so
> much by being taught over here [in the school of

143

nursing], you learn when you actually go and do it on the ward."

"Yeah, I definitely learn on the wards. I mean there are sort of theories of psychology and sociology and there are sort of things you can do in the school but I mean, there's everything you can learn on the ward."

Sometimes, this concept of learning on the wards was compared, not with learning in the school, but with learning from books. It will be noted in the next section, that the student's view of the school or college of nursing was not always complementary. In the following extracts, however, the comparisons are between learning from books and learning in the clinical setting :

"Well, it's alright reading it from a book but actually seeing it on the ward - and actually seeing...like reading about schizophrenia, it is sometimes very difficult to understand unless you actually see a patient displaying thought disorder - like "thought blocking" - then you can understand it much easier, I think."

"Like with medicine. If you did it just by reading books you probably wouldn't remember the tablets and all the different names. When you are on the ward, with a qualified member of staff, you remember them because you can see them in front of you - you can see all the different names on them, not just in a book."

Both of these students were demonstrating the "learning by doing" principle, often encountered in the literature on experiential learning and **described** by the nurse tutors. However, another notable feature was that they talked about learning by "seeing". It would appear that by **seeing** certain elements of nursing, they feel that they are more likely to remember them. This issue is extended to "seeing staff" in the next extract.

"To me, learning by seeing people, to me that's the best way. Actually to see something being applied, practically and then I can develop that. I don't tend to pick things up reading from books but if I go and see

someone being nursed or you read through care plans or
you watch how...what I tend to do is model from senior
nurses if I think they are a good model."

The student, above, demonstrates all of Kolb's stages of the
experiential learning cycle but in the clinical setting. First, she
describes how she has an experience ('seeing something being applied').
The she reflects on what has happened and applies it to another
situation ("and then I can develop that"). She also demonstrates that
she makes an assessment of the nursing staff that she sees around her
and selects one or more out as a "role model". Presumably, though,
she has internalised some criteria for what a "good model" is and it is
interesting to raise the question as to where she came upon such
criteria. She admits that she does not "pick things up reading books";
she also acknowledges that learning about nursing, for her, is best
carried out in the clinical setting. Two possibilities seem likely, here
: a) she has reflected on good practice, herself, and decided upon her
own criteria for what makes a good role model, or b) she has
internalised teaching about good nursing from the school of nursing but
does not make this link explicit.

Sometimes the question of learning in school was explicitly
challenged :

"Me, personally, I probably wouldn't remember as much
if I was learning in the school, if I was in the school all
the time because after so long things tend to go in one
ear and out the other, whereas if you are on the wards
you remember it."

Another student expressed his feelings about the school of
nursing more explicitly :

"Actually, I learn most on the wards. I don't really like
being in school much. Yes, on the wards."

Although "liking being in school" may not be a necessary
condition for learning, this response may be compared to some of the
nurse tutors who stressed that the experiential approach to learning
was an enjoyable one. It seems, for this student, at least, this was not
the case. For one student, too, learning in the school was not so

"real" and no substitute for being in the "real" situation, i.e. the clinical situation :

> "I think learning on the ward, that's the best place you do actually learn. I can remember...we had one of the sisters come over to the school to teach us and we had to actually practice on oranges, which is - when we go out on the wards and actually do it on humans - it's nothing like it. I don't think that even when you practice on an orange, you still haven't learned the technique until you actually do it. I think that goes for an awful lot of things. If you get taught from set to set, from week to week, if you have someone demonstrating to you, well, it isn't actually the same as doing it yourself."

Whilst a number of the tutors felt that they were encouraging the students to practice in a safe setting, it seems that the students often didn't feel that such practice approximated to the "real thing". Permeating all of the student interviews was the theme that the "real thing" was synonymous with "being in the clinical setting".

In the final example in this section, the respondent notes not only the importance of learning in the clinical setting but also a perceived transience of the school learning programme :

> "Well, as I'm on the wards, I have the experience of actually doing the job. You know, when we qualify, or if we qualify, we're not going to be coming back to school ever again, except for things, maybe, like courses. So that what we are really aiming at is for jobs on the wards."

In summary of this section, the feelings and perceptions that permeated most of the students interviews, with respect to the clinical setting and the school of nursing were :
- that when it came to learning about nursing, most of that learning occurred in the clinical setting,
- that the school of nursing was not necessarily an important aspect of their learning process.

Although Fretwell (1982) noted that her research "uncovered aspects of the ward environment which appear to be inconsistent with

146

learning", it is notable that Alexander, in her study of how students learn to nurse (Alexander 1983) was able to recommend that :

>...teachers of nursing [should] teach nursing where nursing is carried out.

In the present study, the evidence, thus far, was that the learners interviewed felt that the clinical setting was the place where they encountered experiential learning.

Experiential Learning in the School or College of Nursing

What, then, were the students' perceptions of the sort of experiential learning that took place in the school or college?   Sometimes, the students' views were very positive and they would have liked more experiential learning in the school or college :

>Respondent :I think it should be a vital part of nurse training and in my view I think that nearly all of our learning should be experiential and I don't think we have enough of it.
>
>Researcher : Which sort are we talking about now...?
>
>Respondent : We're talking about, I think, in the School we should be doing more - more constructive role play. But I find that its not so much. I don't think in the last two years we've ever had a tutor actually recommend or suggest role play.

>"Yeah, well, its quite popular at the moment. Quite the in thing, I suppose. And also because it can work. I think that with certain people, it can work. People can get a lot out of it."

The first respondent, above, felt that nurse tutors should use or recommend role play more often. A clue to why they might not is contained in the next section of this analysis, when students' views of role play are discussed. Not all students enjoyed role play. The second respondent, above, noted the present popularity of experiential learning methods, rather dryly, but also acknowledged their value for "certain people", suggesting, perhaps that experiential learning methods did not suit every student.

On the other hand, some students were unequivocal in their appreciation of the value of experiential learning methods as an approach to "doing" rather than just "listening" :

"They're more important that just sitting down and being told. Its much easier to drum it into you I think if you really experience it."

Another student discriminated between the relative values of certain **types** of experiential learning activities used in the school :

"Some of the counselling techniques that we sort of role played - I can see them going into practice in the ward and I find that they are helpful when I'm on the wards. The icebreakers and things that we do in a group, we tend to do for our pleasure and enjoyment and I don't think we really use them when we're at work."

What is interesting, here, is that a number of tutors commented on the fact that experiential learning activities could be lighthearted and fun to take part in and that they could "make learning enjoyable". This respondent is suggesting that the things that she takes part in that are for her "pleasure and enjoyment" are not things that transfer back to the clinical setting. This, lighter side of experiential learning was commented on by another respondent, thus :

"I think maybe the disadvantage is when you take it as like a comedy at the time. You don't take the serious side of it : you just laugh and joke. You don't think about it seriously and obviously, you're meant to."

This respondent seems clear about the **intention** of the tutor or about the aim of the activities but acknowledges that he or his colleagues can easily find those activities the subject of mirth. It seems, also, that he is suggesting that because of the laughter, the activity is less than useful.

148

Linked to the notion of not taking experiential learning activities seriously was another, perhaps more serious theme : the students view of the school and the tutors in general. Various negative comments were made about the way in which learning sessions were conducted :

> "I wouldn't describe this Nursing School as doing much role play. They usually depend upon the group. They say 'Do you want to do role play?' and if the group say no, then they don't do it."

This appears to be a reference to the ideas suggested by some of the tutors as "negotiating" aspects of the learning process. For this student, however, the negotiation process seems to have broken down and the students' tone (from replaying the interview tape) is one of derogation.

Sometimes, experiential learning and a student centred approach were seen as "easy options" by the students :

> "Well, sometimes its easy for them, sitting down with us. They set you a scene and let you get on with it and they sit back and watch, then tell you what you've done wrong."

A variant on this response was the one offered by this student who felt that the approach to learning lacked structure and clarity :

> "Sometimes its a bit wishy-washy because we're not getting any input at all. You have to do it all yourself. So sometimes you get to a point where you don't really know where you're going..."

Again, it is interesting to compare such responses with the tutors', who claimed that they were breaking down barriers between themselves and the students by being more informal and less structured. It would seem that this was not necessarily the "received" perception. Other respondents were more scathing in their comments about the school and the tutors, although the first of the next group of respondents is reflective about what the tutors were trying to do.

149

"Well, I suppose it's very hard for them to think of things for us to do, you know, or people to invent things, you know. I think its quite sort of a clever idea, really. Well, examples of what we have done, say : you sort of tie your legs together or something or you are blindfolded and someone else has got to lead you around..."

Others, though, were less supportive :

"I don't really learn that much in school. The wards, you remember it because you've got an incident you can put into memory. You don't have to remember which book you were reading and because you are doing it all the time, it becomes easier, doesn't it, as you do more."

"I don't think we get enough input in the school. We are in for one week every three months but sometimes they haven't got the time to teach us."

In the second of the above extracts, it is difficult to know **why** the tutors hadn't got time to teach and the point was not developed by the researcher during the interview.

Sometimes, the complaints about the school and the tutors revolved around the familiar theme of the tutor's being out of date and out of touch with what was happening in the clinical situation :

"To be honest, I feel that everything we've done in the school seems to be a bit irrelevant and sometimes very out dated and I don't feel prepared at all for when I go to a new environment."

"It just that sometimes, it is difficult for them to appreciate this - like the common complaint is that they always forget what its like on the ward once they are in the school. Its difficult for them to appreciate that you haven't just your [school] work : you are working 38 hours a week on the wards."

"Like the staff on the wards say, the tutors should do more, which I think they should come over to the wards more. They don't seem to become involved on the wards and they expect the staff on the wards to do a lot of teaching and they say 'well, we're not teachers : **they've** been trained to teach.'"

"I find the school quite often - this probably sounds like a criticism- but its like they tend not to be living in the real world. OK, all the tutors have worked on the wards before and they are all obviously aware of the situation but, yeah, they set examples in text books and the examples we are given in school have nowhere near the complexity of the person you are dealing with on the ward - just don't even come close."

This last student, above, is not only suggesting that the tutors may be out of date. He is also doing two other things : a) acknowledging those tutors' prior clinical experience (even though that might be out of date) and b) suggesting that the "examples" that tutors use is an oversimplification of real life. This may be an important criticism of some of the experiential learning activities in that they **always** take place away from the "real" situation and therefore, can never exactly match the sort of contingencies that can arise in real life. Another feature of this students' statement is his **apology** : "this probably sounds like a criticism". This sort of apologetic statement was made by a number of students :

"...I know this sounds awful, but..."

"...I know its difficult for them, but..."

Also, the **tone** of the students' comments (through replaying the tapes of the interviews) suggested that some were slightly loath to criticise. Salvage (1985) has noted that nurses work in an atmosphere in which they are not encouraged to be assertive - a point developed by Bond (1986). At least two things may have been happening here : a) the students felt very loyal towards their tutors and felt disloyal in saying negative things about them or b) they had become socialised into the process of **not** saying negative things about senior colleagues.

In closing this section about students perceptions of the school and the tutors, one student, in expressing her dissatisfaction with the experiential learning activities that took place in the school, also

151

recommended her own prescription for how things **might** be. It appears to be very much in line with the theories of experiential learning that advocate learning by direct personal experience :

> "I feel they are very limited in that whenever you are in school it's very difficult to get away from the fact that you are in an artificial environment, you are always aware that it's a game, if you like. They only give you a limited insight whenever you do role play. I would be tempted to say that if I was in charge of education, I would actually sort of send people off to another health authority, have them admitted in to a ward and then actually get the real feel of what its like to come in, because unless you've gone through something yourself, you can't actually have that level of empathy with someone."

This may represent the closest suggestion that any student made about learning through personal experience. The idea of "admitting" students was used as a training device in one school of nursing (Richardson, Bishop et al 1990). In that school, students were asked to spend twenty four hours in a wheelchair in order to experience, as nearly as possible, what it felt like to be profoundly handicapped. Clearly, though, the economics of "admitting" every student to another hospital is unlikely to make the suggestion a particularly practical one.

Just as some of the tutors were worried about whether or not students would feel "safe" taking part in experiential learning activities, a number of students expressed their anxieties in this area. Some admitted to feeling considerably less than emotionally safe and the lack of safety often surrounded the issue of self-disclosure. Talking of a particular learning session in a school of nursing, one student suggested that :

> "I think that they felt as if they had exposed something that they didn't want to expose : they had been exposed to the group...I just think its wrong for people to be so distressed if they don't want to be, in front of everyone else."

Others also talked about the painful process of the process of either 'breaking down' or of self-disclosure :

> "Well, I think people can be upset, breaking down in front of everybody...it shouldn't get to that stage."

Sometimes this discomfort was linked to the issue of **voluntariness** or the freedom to elect not to take part in an experiential learning activity :

> " I think, sometimes if you go into a session and you don't know what you are doing, it can be quite threatening. If somebody explains to you what you are going to do before hand, and also the fact that if we don't want to do it, we don't have to - I mean, we can just sit and observe."

> "Well. we're all sitting round in a group and we were not told what we're doing and we're not given the option to opt out if we want and you don't know what's going to happen. I don't like that."

Heron (1989a) suggests that **all** experiential learning activities should be entered into freely. As adults, students should be free to decide, beforehand, whether or not a suggested activity will suit them and whether or not they wish to take part. Such a "voluntary clause" as Heron has called it (Heron 1977b) is problematic. First, it cannot be assumed that just because a tutor tells a group of students that they can "sit out" if they wish, that they will exercise their right to do that. Group pressure, peer pressure and the hierarchial relationship between tutor and student may all mitigate against students choosing freely in this way - despite the fact that many of the tutors in this study wanted a "more equal" relationship with their students. None of the students mentioned this "more equal" relationship. It may be easier to throw off status when you are in a higher status position than it is to throw it off if you are in a lower status position.

Also, on the issue of voluntariness, there is no way for the students to anticipate what may happen in any given activity. If an exercise or activity is likely to provoke an emotional response (and many of the ones in the literature are aimed at the affective domain), then it may be difficult for students to know what they will feel like once they have started the exercise. They may a) not know that they are allowed to withdraw from the activity once it has started or b) be unable to control their emotions once they have been stirred up. It would appear that **structure** of experiential learning activities may be a factor here. One student reported as follows :

> "Groups - you can learn about yourself from groups but at the same time its got to be under structure because everybody's really frightened about disclosing anything and very defensive."

The questions of structure and control were developed by another student who put it this way :

> "When we have done role play, if we've been taking personal situations, we've always had tutors who could control the situation. I mean, things can get out of control. We've always had the option, you know, if you don't want to, you don't have to. So if you don't want to divulge any information, its been OK in my experience."

Again, Heron (1977b) suggests that structure, particularly in the early stages of group development in educational settings, can help people to feel more secure and give them a sense of personal control. It would seem that the students in this study had mixed views about whether or not **their** tutors where able to develop such structure. On the other hand, many of the **tutors** expressed the view that they merely set up a variety of activities and waited to see what happened. As we shall see, not all of the students responded well to this approach. An experiential learning activity that was frequently discussed (and frequently discussed in a negative light) was role play. It is on role play that attention is now focused.

Role Play

The student group could be divided into those who liked role play and those who did not : there were few "in betweens". The largest group was those who did not like it. First, the students who liked it and

154

found it useful. Sometimes, there was a straightforward acknowledgement of it as a learning technique :

"Well, I like role play. I don't think there is a limit to the practical things you can do with it."

"I enjoy it. I enjoy it very much."

"Well it does sort of reproduce a sort of situation that could happen on the ward. It does make you think of how to put things into practice. What we have learned, sort of like communication skills, body space, posture : so it does sort of help in that it is a less severe atmosphere than on the ward."

"I think role plays were good actually. This was sort of very embarrassing to do, but once you get used to it, I think its once of the most important exercises that we do."

All of these students were able to make a link between doing the role play and that role play's value as an educational experience. The third respondent, above, makes explicit reference to how certain interpersonal skills, learnt in the school of nursing could be carried over into the clinical setting via such role play.

Sometimes, though, there was a "but" acknowledged in the student's response. Often, this took the form of "I like it but I know students who don't."

"I enjoy role play but some people just don't like doing it because they have to put themselves in role positions, they have to see another point of view. They might be quite an immature type of person."

"In my group, they shy away from it, role play exercises, saying its silly, things like that. There's only really two of us in the group who do enjoy it and get a lot out of doing role play because we actually try to put ourselves in that position : whereas the others don't really get themselves into that position so I don't think they benefit from it much."

155

In the first of these cases, there is a judgement that people who don't like role play may be immature. In both of the quotations, there is a suggestion that what other people find difficult about role play is the 'putting yourself in someone else's position'. This seem allied to empathy, which has been described as being able to enter the frame of reference of another person (Rogers 1967). Also, Rogers suggested that empathy was one of the necessary and sufficient factors in therapeutic change (Rogers 1957). Recent research, however, suggests that empathy is a loosely defined concept and neither easily measured nor easily classified as such an important concept that it can be counted as a necessary and sufficient ingredient of a therapeutic relationship (Mackay and Carvar 1990). This empathising aspect of role play was noted by another student who liked role play :

"I enjoy role play, but I have found in our set and with a lot of other sets I see doing it, there are people very reluctant to do it. I enjoy it. I feel I learn a lot from it because, you know, role play - you can put yourself in that person's position and see what it was like for them, from their point of view."

The question of learning about empathy and other interpersonal skills, such as counselling was discussed by another student in a largely positive light :

'It's artificial in a way, but if you are talking particularly about counselling situations, it is one way of learning to deal with people or talk to people. Role play exercises are good in that way, but then again, its artificial in a way that its a story - its not real - but its a way of picking up techniques, counselling techniques.

Despite the acknowledgement of the "artificiality" of the role play situation, the student found role play a useful way to learn counselling methods.

Another student felt that the **idea** of role play was a good one but that it was not sufficiently or appropriately used. She suggested how it may be made more appropriate to clinical nursing :

156

"Maybe it would be a good idea whereby you do the role play here [in the school] and you do a little bit of it then your expected to carry it on to the patients, without supervision, but will, like, be sitting in a room where the tutor will be. Then, maybe, it would be the right atmosphere then, when the tutors come over on the ward. I think one day a week or something, so that the students on the ward could have a role play session. But we should do it **there** [in the clinical setting] because its nothing to do with the school."

This student seemed to be acknowledging a variety of things. First, she seemed to feel that role play could be useful (in that she was suggesting its use at all). More than that, however, she was seeing it as a possible way of integrating the tutorial staff from the school of nursing into the clinical setting. It is almost as though she was offering it as an "excuse" for the tutors to visit the wards - that it offered them a definite role in the clinical setting. She noted, too, that role play had "nothing to do with the school".

Returning to the issue of why some people did not like role play, we return to the issues of being able to "act", to take on the role of another person. A number of students felt that the "acting" aspect of the role play made them either embarrassed or made them doubt the value of the role play on the grounds that it was "artificial". One student **appreciated** the artificial aspect and saw it as a positive and educational factor :

"When I do role play in the classroom, everybody's aware that it's a false situation and maybe an ideal situation so it's good, in a way, to feel that you can make mistakes in the classroom and it doesn't really matter."

Others, though, were less certain of the value of it and found that the embarrassment and unreality factors seemed to get in the way. Often, too, they supported the idea that role play appealed to certain sorts of people : often more extrovert people than themselves.

"Well, people who don't mind performing in front of a group like it. I would say, generally, that more extrovert people like it."

157

'Well, role play is embarrassing : standing up in front of everyone else, you know, and having to do something. Whereas if you sit and do something slightly more practical, if everybody's doing it, then the spotlight isn't on you.'

"I think its too much of a false situation. I try to sit and watch with other people and learn a bit from it but I don't do it myself. I'll do other things, but not specifically role play."

"I think role play is OK if you feel comfortable doing it but personally I fell silly doing it so I don't do it now."

The last two respondents, in suggesting that they 'don't do it' imply that they have **choice** in whether or not they take part. Also, the first of those two suggests that she learns vicariously, by watching others doing role play. The second respondent, above, seems to be highlighting the need not to be "put on the spot" but to be allowed to feel part of the group. The issues of choice and of different teaching and learning methods suiting different people was taken up by another student :

"I just know that some people say "I don't like role play, I'd rather not do it." And since it's generally a voluntary thing you are not held to do this or that or the other. Maybe its because they don't think that role play is of any value in learning. Some people very much like the conventional teaching approach and think that the only kind of proper teaching is where they have got somebody sort of telling them a list of facts and then writing it down. Some people are happier with that. I don't think that's a kind of criticism or them. That's just : people have different preferences."

Here, then, role play was being compared to more "traditional" learning and teaching methods : an allusion made by a number of the nurse tutors. The respondent also suggested that various methods may suit different people, even though his comments about some people thinking that the "only kind of proper teaching" involves listening and taking notes, **seemed** to contain a negative evaluation of such people.

Some students, however, were quite clear that role play was not an approach that they like or that suited them :

"I don't like role play."

"The fact that it is not for real and that you are acting. That's the thing I don't like."

It is interesting to compare these frequent suggestions of the unreality of role play with the same students' citing of clinical learning as 'real'. It seemed that for many of the students, the real situation **was** the clinical situation and rehearsing or role playing clinical possibilities seemed like a poor imitation of the real thing. Also, in summary, it appeared that students who were more extrovert and able to self-disclose easily where more likely to benefit from and enjoy role play. The "make believe" element of role play, turned out not to appeal to "younger" students. Perhaps this could be attributed to the age factor. Perhaps it is necessary for students who are still making the transition from childhood, through late adolescence and into adulthood, to experience a stage where they do not have to do anything that they consider "childish" (such as "pretending" or "play acting"). In support of this suggestion, more of the tutors felt comfortable with role play than did students.

On the other hand, such tutors would also be **in control** of the role play and in a dominant position vis a vis the students. The educator's role could be compared to that of "director" and this label has been used explicitly by Moreno (1959, 1969, 1977) in his writings on psychodrama. The role of director may be a powerful one in that a director make suggestions about what others might do. This, it would appear, may suit tutors more than it does students. Ironically, too, if tutors **do** adopt this director role, it returns them to a situation in which they are **prescriptive** in their relationships with students - despite many of them suggesting that they would prefer a more equal relationship with those students. Overall, it appeared that the tutors where much more in favour of using role play as an experiential learning method than were the students.

Experiential Learning Methods

For the sake of completeness, it is useful to note the sorts of experiential learning methods that students said that they had taken part in. A wide range of exercises and activities were identified by the students and that range covered most of the activities described in the literature as "experiential learning methods" and those described by the tutors.

"We have had role play, small group exercises, empathy exercises, ice-breakers, games, those sorts of things."

"We have done other things like being blindfolded and tied up and so forth and we've done role play and psychodrama."

"We've done psychodrama and lots of exercises."

These quotations represent what many of the students repeated: that they had taken part in a wide range of activities that could be called "experiential learning activities".

Advantages of Experiential Learning and Articulating What Experiential Learning Is

A number of the students made links between the various approaches to experiential learning in the school of nursing and the value of those approaches in terms of the clinical setting.

"For me, it [experiential learning] linked up in a way that I can develop counselling techniques. Although artificially, I can develop techniques, judge situations, body language, posture, tone of voice, putting yourself in an artificial situation stimulates response and that useful and helps me in the ward."

Here, the acknowledgement was made that the activities used produced an "artificial" situation but that situation was both useful and clinically applicable. On a similar but different note, some students found the use of blindfolds to simulate blindness and

160

activities in which they were encouraged to imagine what it was like to hallucinate, or be handicapped useful, as it made them reconsider their attitudes and feelings towards blindness, schizophrenia and disablement. They were able to describe their progress through these such activities :

"I think as far as the blindfolding was concerned - I think sort of actually telling, actually teaching a class of nursing, telling them what its like to be blind - I still don't think you can appreciate it, what its like. I suppose being blindfolded is really putting you in the situation to some extent. It's then that you really appreciate what it;s like and really empathise....It's like the same for schizophrenia and things. You know this person is hearing voices and you've no experience what its like and you have to counsel that person, perhaps. But actually sitting there with earphones on and having a voice whisper to you just shows that it can be frightening. It modifies your attitude to a great extent, that sort of exercise. I mean, actual formal teaching isn't so likely to modify that."

"The empathy exercises we had I thought were good, actually, because we did exercises where we were actually blindfolded. We had an arm in a sling and you had to be led around for quite a while by another member. Yes, it did make, give you an understanding or what it must be like being blind or handicapped in some way. So I thought those exercises were very good."

Some difference may be noted between the above "simulations" and role play. In the simulations referred to above, the students were put in a situation, by the use of "props" to help them to experience sensory or motor deprivation. In role play, however, they were asked to **play** another person. In the former situation, the students were helped to experience the world from another person's point of view through active intervention on the part of the tutors. In the role play situation, the students had to **imagine** what another person's world might be like. Arguably, the more concrete 'simulation' allowed for a more dramatic appreciation of other people's lives. Also, the simulation encouraged the students to undertake stages in Kolb's

(1984) experiential learning cycle, discussed in the first chapter. They were offered an experience (eg being blindfolded) they then reflected on that experience and then carried the learning over into the "real" situation. In one case, above, the student felt that this had "modified your attitude" and noted that the **doing** of this activity was more likely to produce such attitude change than would more traditional, formal teaching. This issue of "experiencing" was taken up by another student :

> "If you learn about something and you actually experience it, then that's when it sinks it. In the same way if you have a piece of research to do rather than picking up a book and reproducing it verbatim, you actually go out an experience the research yourself. That's the way that you learn and it's more beneficial in that way because you are actually going through the situation."

The "going through the situation" may be the key to the students' perceptions of learning and remembering. Throughout the interviews students frequently referred to learning in the clinical setting rather than in the school of college of nursing. Others, as we have noted, thought that "seeing" a situation made much more sense to them than reading about it or "being taught" about it. Given that the major part of the life-world of the student is the clinical setting and given the frequent suggestions by them that "doing" is better that "being taught" it would seem that experiential learning as perceived by the students has much to do with learning by being personally involved and immersed in the learning situation : being **active** rather than **passive** learners. A number of students tried to put this into words :

> "Well, I suppose it makes you look at things in a different way, you know. An experience, I suppose. Well, its not learning as in remembering, its just : I suppose you remember what you've experienced **better**. You apply it, perhaps. No, you can apply it because it means more to you, perhaps."

For this student, capturing the essence of what experience meant was not easy but he seemed to be conveying this sense of the primacy of experience itself, rather than having just "remembered" things. Another student developed this theme in a personalised way. He saw experiential learning as concerned with "personal knowledge" rather in the way that it was discussed in the first chapter :

> "You'd be involved more as an individual person. Nobody else would have your knowledge, your skills, because its **you** view on a particular subject; its **your** view on say, psychology. If you are looking at a particular subject and you read that, then you develop **your own** views and your own particular perspective."

Another student was able to distinguish between this process of learning from personal experience and another domain of "factual knowledge":

> "I think, as with the case of the blindfold, you might know someone who's blind and perhaps your own previous life experience may influence your reaction to it perhaps. I think you do need, as well as learning from experience, you do need the sort of factual backup from the school, the theory."

This student seems to be acknowledging the **limitations** of personal experience and suggesting that theoretical and factual knowledge are important alongside the more personal or experiential knowledge (Heron 1981).

It is here that we have come full circle. It will be noted in this analysis, that students often began by describing experiential learning as learning in the clinical setting, in the "real world". Here, in closing, we see that view confirmed and enlarged a little to take account of experiential learning being personal learning, learning by doing and learning by being involved in what is happening, as opposed to "traditional" textbook, school or "remembering things" learning. Some of the things that distinguish the student's view of experiential learning from the educator's view, is that the tutors tended to elaborate the concept of experiential learning with reference to "philosophies of teaching and learning"- particularly the humanistic philosophy. The students appeared to take a more pragmatic view : "I learn things by doing them". Also, the tutors tended to emphasise the role of self-awareness and self-disclosure in the learning process,

163

whilst the students were quite often embarrassed by such issues and preferred to choose their own rate of self-disclosure.

In the final chapter of this book, the similarities and differences between the two groups are pulled together. First, however, it is necessary to explore how a larger group of tutors and students viewed experiential learning via a questionnaire generated out of the data so far collected.

Further Validation

The problems of validating qualitative research are various. How do you know that you have managed to "bracket" your own beliefs, values and attitudes? Who is to say that your analysis of the data is a reasonable or accurate one? What other interpretations could be made of the data? One way of attempting to validate findings from qualitative data is to invite respondents to review the analysis and for them to identify the degree to which they do or do not "agree" with that analysis. This, too, is fraught. The problems identified, above, are problems for the **reviewer** in exactly the same way as they are for the researcher. Bloor (1978) reported that when he asked his respondents to check his findings, some findings were agreed but the respondents also identified a range of **other** findings. For Abrahams (1984) the situation was worse. He reported that his validation project "turned into a series of furious arguments, wrangles and recriminations". The task of attempting validation was therefore approached with some trepidation.

It was decided that, as earlier stages of the interview analyses had been checked with respondents during the various stages of analysis, the researcher would invite one respondent to read through all of the analyses and findings and comment on them. This was following Ball's (1984) approach, when he invited a respondent to read various drafts and chapters of his research report. A respondent was found who was also involved in research in the social sciences although in an entirely different field. After reading the analysis, there was a long a detailed discussion over the categories and analyses. Overall, the respondent "agreed" with those categories and analyses although he would have liked to have seen more made of the issue of the "transfer of learning" issue. Small modification were made to some of the names of the categories, but, overall, the analysis remained as it was. However, the **process** of discussing the analyses with another person proved useful in considering how to develop the questionnaire in the next section. The discussion also served as a further means of helping to ensure the validity of the research process being undertaken.

Conclusion

In summary, it can be said that the students tended to view experiential learning in clinical and practical terms. They also saw it as a personal and active approach to learning and one that may not be popular if it involved role play. The students also noted a divide between clinical learning on the one hand and "school" learning on the other.

8   The wider field: A survey of experiential learning

This chapter explores the second stage of the research project and describes :

- The questionnaire design,
- The sample,
- Access,
- Distribution of the questionnaire,
- Analysis of the questionnaire.

Introduction

Following the interviews and the analysis of the data that evolved, the second stage of the project developed : the survey of a larger sample of tutors and students through the use of a questionnaire.   This chapter describes and discusses that second stage.

Second Stage of the Research Project

The previous chapters have described how a picture of the perceptions of 12 nurse tutors and 12 student nurses, with regard to experiential learning was built up. It has also described how two forms of analysis were used to examine the data collected - first through a relatively straightforward content analysis and frequency count and second, through a more detailed qualitative analysis. In the second stage of the study, a questionnaire was developed from these findings and distributed to a larger sample.

Questionnaire Design

Once the transcripts had been analysed using the two approaches described above, certain clear themes began to emerge. These were described in previous chapters. Using these themes, a questionnaire was developed in order to check the degree to which a larger sample of tutors and students did or did not support the findings obtained during the interviews. The questionnaire sought to obtain the following information :

- the ways in which nurse tutors and students **defined** experiential learning,
- the sorts of experiential learning methods they had experienced, either as teachers or as students,
- nurse tutors' and students' beliefs about the nature of nurse education and experiential learning as discussed by the previous sample of 24,
- nurse tutors' and students' perceptions of experiential learning,
- certain demographic data.

The questionnaire was developed through discussion with colleagues and through a reading of some of the literature on questionnaire design (e.g. Oppenheim 1966, Treece and Treece 1977, Youngman 1978, Couchman and Dawson 1990). The questionnaire was also shown to colleagues who were asked to play a "devil"s advocate" role in order to attempt to weed out the obviously problematic items. In the end, a questionnaire containing a mixture of biographical questions, questions about experiential learning methods and some Likert - type questions (Moser and Kalton 1971) which enabled the exploration of beliefs about nurse education and experiential learning.

167

The principles that governed the production of the questionnaire were as follows :

- the questionnaire should not be too long, to ensure a reasonable return,
- the wording of it should not be ambiguous,
- it should obtain information from both nurse tutors and students.
- the items in the questionnaire should reflect issues discussed by the students and nurse tutors in the interviews conducted earlier.

Face Validity

The questionnaire was assessed by a panel of experts comprised of professors of nursing from two universities, a lecturer in nursing studies with experience of questionnaire design and a statistician. The aim was to check the degree to which the questionnaire both represented issues identified during the previous interviews of students and nurse tutors and to check that it offered a reasonable means of identifying a further group of students' and tutors' perceptions of experiential learning. Checking for face validity is identified as an essential feature of questionnaire design by Kidder and Judd (1986).

Following comments from the panel of experts, the questionnaire was modified to reflect their comments which had mostly to do with the ordering of the questions and with the position of the three sections of the questionnaire (1. experiential learning methods, 2. perceptions of nurse education and experiential learning and 3. demographic information). The pilot study process was also a means of helping to establish face validity.

Pilot Study

The questionnaire was piloted using a group of 15 nurse tutors and 20 student nurses from schools of nursing in England and that were not being included in the sample used for the survey. 30 questionnaires were returned, coded and analysed. Respondents were asked to comment on the questionnaire design and the ease (or otherwise) of its completion. Following this pilot study, minor modifications were made to various questions to reduce ambiguity. Also, the order of presentation of some questions was changed in order that there should not be too much overlap of topic.

The problem of the halo effect is always present in questionnaire design (Oppenheim 1966). The respondent may adopt an overall feeling of like or dislike towards the general topic of the questionnaire and answer according to that overall disposition, rather than addressing each item with a relatively open mind. An attempt to counteract this effect was made at the post-pilot stage by varying the position of some of the "negative" and "positive" questions. The person who is influenced by the halo effect will sometimes spot an apparent trend or pattern in the questionnaire layout and continue marking down one side of the page, with little stopping to check how the questions **actually** read. The breaking up of any "patterns" of questions can help to counteract this.

Overall, the format of the questionnaire proved to be satisfactory and copies of the final draft were produced for use with the identified sample. The pilot study process also helped to clarify the best way of coding the questionnaire.

Sample

The decision was taken to use the schools of nursing in Wales as the total population for the second part of the study. Wales is a discrete Principality containing health districts with schools and colleges of nursing of different sorts. It therefore allowed for variety of location and types of schools. Also, those schools are separated by considerable distance, thus allowing, again for variation in philosophy of training and care.

The Welsh National Board for Nursing, Midwifery and Health Visiting was approached for details of the student and tutor population in Wales but were unable to give exact figures of nursing in training. Therefore, each director of nurse education in each of the eight areas of training in Wales was written to and asked for details of their total numbers of tutors and students in general nursing and psychiatric nursing. This population is illustrated in Table 8.1.

Table 8.1

Total Populations :

Tutors and Students, General and Psychiatric Nursing, Wales,
January 1990

General and Psychiatric nurse tutors in post, in Wales, January 1990.	184
General and Psychiatric nursing students in post, in Wales, January 1990.	3250

From these figures, it was decided to survey all of the general nursing and psychiatric nursing tutors (184) and 10% of the general and 10% of the psychiatric nursing students in training (325). Other specialties, such as mental handicap nursing and childrens nursing were excluded from the sample because of the small numbers involved.

Table 8.2

Total Sample for Questionnaire Distribution

All Nurse Tutors in general and psychiatric schools of nursing in Wales, January 1990	184
10% of student nurses in general and psychiatric nurse training, in Wales, January 1990	325

The total sampling frame is illustrated in Table 8.2. The type of sample can be described as a stratified sample (Kidder and Judd 1986, Pilcher 1990). Given the geography of the Principality and the relatively large distances between the various schools and colleges, it was decided to conduct a postal questionnaire. The most obvious limitation of this approach is that it tends to lead to a less complete return than does the personal administration of questionnaires by the researcher (Oppenheim 1969, Kidder and Judd 1986). This problem was offset by the fact that the researcher was able to contact many of the directors of nurse education and senior tutors by phone. This personal approach seemed to pay dividends in that a good response to the survey was obtained.

It will be noted, from the discussion above, that the sample of nurse tutors and tutors was a **total** one. The sample of students involved making decisions about how those students should be selected for the survey.

The issue of randomness in a sample is a fraught one. On the one hand, for a sample to be truly random, each person in the total population must stand an equal chance of being included in the selected sample population. In this case, this would have meant the researcher being able to have access to the names and addresses of all of the students in training at a particular time and then his using a table of random numbers (or similar means) to obtain a random sample. In practice, the Welsh National Board for Nursing, Midwifery and Health Visiting was not able to furnish such a list. Also, as an education officer from that office pointed out, the population of students in training at any given time is constantly fluctuating. It is also important to note that the sample was used to generate **descriptive** data. There was no intention to generalise the findings to a total population of tutors and students in the UK.

In order to increase the representative nature of the sample, no attempt was made to influence which groups of students were selected to complete the questionnaire in the eight areas. The nurse tutors responsible for the training and education of those students were asked to ask groups of students that were studying in the school at the time of receipt of the questionnaires, to complete them. In this way a degree of chance was introduced in that students could thus be from any year of training and not specially "selected" by any particular criteria except that of the students' being in school at the time. At all times, the principle of voluntariness was observed : both tutors and students were free not to take part in the survey if they so chose.

Access to Sample

A "top down" approach to gaining access to both tutors and students was used. The eight directors of nurse educator were approached by letter for access to the next level of responsibility : senior tutors. Once permission was obtained from those directors, permission was sought from senior tutors to send questionnaires to tutors and for a tutor to distribute questionnaires to groups of students.

In one health authority, it was policy that all requests to collect data from both patients and staff be considered by a nursing ethics

171

committee. In this case, a detailed protocol was sent to that committee and permission granted for the approaches to tutors and students to be made.

Distribution of the Questionnaire

Senior tutors in the eight health authorities were contacted by phone and asked if they would be prepared to circulate the questionnaires amongst their tutorial staff and to a group of students of any year. All senior tutors were agreeable to cooperating in this way and the questionnaires were sent by post, along with a stamped addressed envelopes for their return. A covering letter was sent with each batch of questionnaires affirming that no student or school would be named in the final report and asking that the questionnaires be returned by a particular date, usually two and a half weeks following the sending out of the questionnaire. Naming a date for return is suggested as a way of helping to ensure a prompt return of postal questionnaires (Youngman 1978).

Return

Completed questionnaire were returned fairly promptly by most correspondents. To encourage a further return, a follow up letter was sent to all correspondents five weeks after the initial set of questionnaires had been sent out. The response rate was 77.9 % which can be seen as a reasonably good response. Oppenheim (1966) points out that :

> For respondents who have no special interest in the subject matter of the [postal] questionnaire, figures of 40 per cent to 60 per cent are typical; even in studies of interested groups, 80 per cent is seldom exceeded. (Oppenheim 1966 : 34)

The response rate could be attributed to a number of factors. First, a number of the senior tutors contacted by the researcher either knew the researcher by acquaintance or by name. Second, the questionnaire was relatively short and easy to complete. Dillman (1978) noted that questionnaires over about 12 pages in length tend to lead to a decreased response rate. Youngman (1978) also noted that a well designed and produced questionnaire tends to encourage a good response rate. Third, the questionnaires that were distributed to students were likely to be distributed to any group of students that were in the school or college at the time of receipt by the tutors concerned. This may have prompted the tendency to deal with the questionnaire quickly in order to "clear the desk" of them. Also, the return envelopes were of the self-addressed, stamped variety, with the return address having been written on the envelope by the researcher. Scott (1961) noted that these tend to secure a higher return rate than do business reply envelopes. He also reports that interest in the subject matter of the questionnaire by the respondents tends to secure a higher return rate.

The issue of whether or not the senior tutors (who distributed the questionnaires to their students and tutors) knew or knew of the researcher is a difficult one. One the one hand, it seems possible that such knowledge of the researcher and his interest in experiential learning might bias responses in particular instances. On the other, such knowledge might "cancel itself out" in the following way. First, if a particular respondent felt that he or she "agreed" with any views expressed in publications by the researcher and sought to express this in his or her response, then it seems possible that others would seek to show "disagreement" in the same way. Also, it is argued that the researcher has expressed a **variety** of views about experiential learning in publications on the topic (Burnard 1985, 1986, 1987a, 1988a, 1989c). Further, it seems likely that only **tutors** responses were likely to be affected in this way (if, indeed, they were) : students were possibly less likely to have reviewed the literature on experiential learning. In the end, the issue is an impossible one to deal with through conventional research methods. Presumably the only way to have ensured a "clean" response would have been for the researcher to adopt an assumed name. This, in turn, may have affected the good response rate.

Method of Analysis

On return of the questionnaires, each was coded by hand by allocating a number to each of the items in the questionnaire. Thus, in the first part of the questionnaire (the part concerning the experiential learning methods that respondents had either used or taken part in, the figure

I was marked alongside a tick or positive response to the item, or a figure O was marked to indicate that no tick or positive response was present.

The second part of the questionnaire required that the respondents answer either STRONGLY AGREE, AGREE, UNCERTAIN, DISAGREE, or STRONGLY DISAGREE with a series of statements. This section was coded as follows :

- If a STRONGLY AGREE response was present, the figure 5 was allocated to that response,
- If an AGREE response was present, the figure 4 was allocated,
- IF an UNCERTAIN response was present, the figure 3 was allocated,
- If a DISAGREE response was present, the figure 2 was allocated,
- If a STRONGLY DISAGREE response was present, the figure 1 was allocated,
- If a response to any item was missing, the figure 9 was allocated. This was used to ensure consistent coding of each item throughout each questionnaire.

In the final section of the questionnaire, demographic data was sought.

In order to facilitate the reading of the "raw" data, a codebook was developed that helped to identify which code number referred to which item of the questionnaire.

Once all the questionnaires had been coded, those codes were entered onto a datasheet - a grid which prepares the data for entry onto disc for use with the computer version of SPSS. Thus a fairly large dataset was developed. This dataset was then entered into the mainframe computer system of the University of Wales College of Medicine by the computing department of that institution and downloaded onto floppy disc for use with the SPSS/PC software package.

The SPSS/PC software package is a personal computer version of the well known Statistics Package for Social Scientists, which had previously been available for use on mainframe computers. The PC version was used by the researcher to compute frequency counts of various aspects of the questionnaire, including :

- Characteristics of the sample,

- Numbers and types of experiential learning methods used or taken part in by respondents,
- Responses to the Likert-type questions.

Using the software package entailed learning how to use the program and identifying the particular requirements for this project. The SPSS/PC program is a large and powerful one and is capable of running a variety of statistical tests on data. What had to be borne in mind at all times were the following characteristics of the data :

- The differences in **type** of sample. Whilst the tutor sample was a total one, the student sample was a 10% one that, although stratified, was not random.
- There were differences in the numbers in each sample group : there were 325 students and 184 tutors.
- There were differences in the type of data obtained. The first part of the questionnaire asked for "yes" or "no" answers to whether or not respondents had experience of a variety of types of experiential learning methods. Thus, this section of the questionnaire produced **nominal** data. The second section invited respondents to rate their perceptions on a five-point scale, thus producing **ordinal** data.

It was important, therefore, to proceed with caution when attempting to apply any statistical tests to such data. It borne in mind that the **aim** was to produce a **description** of some tutors' and students' perceptions of experiential learning.

Stages in the Analysis of the Data

The following stages were worked through in analysing the data obtained from the questionnaire. It was found helpful to identify exactly what was could be collated from the data set in an organised manner before the SPSS/PC package was used. In this way the researcher was able to avoid becoming lost in both the data set and the computer program.

Stage One : Demographic Details

The following characteristics of the sample were computed :
- Total student response,
- Total tutor response,

- Numbers of general and psychiatric students,
- Numbers of general and psychiatric tutors,
- Age ranges of the general and psychiatric students,
- Age ranges of the general and psychiatric tutors.

Stage Two : Experiential Learning Methods

The following were identified from the data :
- Total frequency counts for each method, by student,
- Total frequency counts for each method, by tutors,
- Frequency counts for general and psychiatric students,
- Frequency counts for general and psychiatric tutors.

Stage Three : Likert-type Data

From the middle section of the questionnaire, in which respondents were asked to identify their perceptions using a five-point scale, the following sub-stages were worked through.
- Frequency counts were identified for the total sample, thus identifying counts within the categories "strongly agree". "agree", "uncertain", disagree" and "strongly disagree". Following this first count, it was decided to collapse the responses," "agree" and "strongly agree"" and " "disagree" and "strongly disagree"" as few responses fell in the "strong" categories.
- Frequency counts were identified for the total sample, the student group and the educator group, using the categories, "agree", "uncertain" and "disagree". Further frequency counts were then computed for the general student, psychiatric student, general tutor and psychiatric tutor groups.
- The findings from these counts were converted into percentages so that the student and educator groups could be compared.
- The responses to the "agree" category for the total sample, the student group and the educator groups were rank ordered, by percentage, thus allowing for the development of a chart for comparison of the findings. Following the rank order of the items according to an analysis of all of the respondents" "agree" statements, the values for the student and tutors

176

groups were placed alongside this rank order list. In this way, comparisons could be made of the various groups. An illustration may clarify this part of the process. Figure 8.1. illustrates part of the first rank ordering, by "all respondents".

RANK ORDER	STATEMENT	ALL RESPONDENTS % (n=397)
1.	Experiential learning can be fun.	92
2.	Student nurses learn best from personal experience.	91

Figure 8.1 : Part of the first stage of rank ordering by "all" agree statements, by percentage

Following this initial rank ordering, the percentages for the student and tutor groups were added to each of the items, as illustrated in figure 8.2. It should be borne in mind what is being illustrated here. The "all" category represents the percentages of the **total respondent sample** who answered "agree" to each item. The "general tutor" category represents the percentage of the **general tutor** sample and so on. Thus, it is quite possible to have values in the tutor and student groups which are considerably higher or lower than the average for "all". Given that each tutor and student group contained different numbers of respondents, the only point of comparison was through percentages.

RANK ORDER	STATEMENTS	A %	GT %	PT %	GS %	PS %
1.	Experiential learning can be fun.	92	95	89	91	90
2.	Student nurses learn best from personal experience.	91	86	89	94	85

KEY :

A = All respondents (n=397)
GT = General tutors (n=109)
PT = Psychiatric tutors (n=26)
GS = General students (n=222)
PS = Psychiatric students (n=40)

Figure 8.2. Part of the elaborated rank order list, showing columns for the tutor and student group averages

• Once the full chart of "agree" responses was developed, it was possible to identify similarities and differences between responses. By careful scrutiny of the chart, it was possible to identify certain patterns in the data. These patterns were identified using the following method of analysis.

Method of Analysis of the Rank Order List

A series of categories was developed so that all of the items in the rank order list could be accounted for. The paragraphs that follow identify those categories and show the criteria used to include statements within each category.

Category 1   Experiential Learning : The Overall View

Nature of the Category : The statements in this category represented items that most of the respondents were in agreement with both at a high level of agreement and at a low level.

178

A. High Level of Agreement With Statements

Criterion for Inclusion : Responses where tutors and students of all groups were in general agreement with a statement at a level not less than 82%.

EXAMPLE

RANK	STATEMENT	A %	GT %	PT %	GS %	PS %
1.	Experiential learning can be fun.	92	95	89	91	90

Key : A = All respondents (n=397)
   GT = General nurse tutors (n=109)
   PT = Psychiatric nurse tutors (n=26)
   GS = General nurse students (n=222)
   PS = Psychiatric nurse students (n=40)

B. Low Level of Agreement with Statements

Criterion for Inclusion : Responses where tutors and students of all groups were in accord regarding agreement with a statement at a low level (single figure percentages). In other words, these were the statements that were most strongly disagreed with.

EXAMPLE

RANK	STATEMENT	A %	GT %	PT %	GS %	PS %
36.	Experiential learning methods suit all teachers.	4	6	4	3	4

Key : A = All respondents (n=397)
    GT = General nurse tutors (n=109)
    PT = Psychiatric nurse tutors (n=26)
    GS = General nurse students (n=222)
    PS = Psychiatric nurse students (n=40)

Category 2 The Tutors View

Nature of the Category : The statements in this category were items that illustrated the tutors' viewpoint (both general and psychiatric tutors).
Criterion for Inclusion : Responses where there was a higher level of agreement to a statement in both tutor groups when compared to both student groups.

EXAMPLE

RANK	STATEMENT	A %	GT %	PT %	GS %	PS %
9.	Experiential learning methods do not suit all learners.	80	85	85	78	80

Key : A = All respondents (n=397)
    GT = General nurse tutors (n=109)
    PT = Psychiatric nurse tutors (n=26)
    GS = General nurse students (n=222)
    PS = Psychiatric nurse students (n=40)

Category 3 The Students View

Nature of the Category : The statements in this category were items that illustrated the students' viewpoint (both general and psychiatric students).

Criterion for Inclusion : Responses where there was a higher level of agreement to a statement in both student groups when compared to both student groups.

EXAMPLE

RANK	STATEMENT	A %	GT %	PT %	GS %	PS %
26.5	Experiential learning methods are easy to take part in.	41	21	12	53	44

Key : A = All respondents (n=397)
   GT = General nurse tutors (n=109)
   PT = Psychiatric nurse tutors (n=26)
   GS = General nurse students (n=222)
   PS = Psychiatric nurse students (n=40)

Category 4 The Psychiatric Tutors View

Nature of the Category : The statements in this category were items that represented the psychiatric tutors' viewpoint.

Criterion for Inclusion : Responses where there was a higher level of agreement to a statement by psychiatric nurse tutors than by any of the other groups and where there was an at least 5% higher rating by the psychiatric tutors than the next nearest category of respondents.

EXAMPLE

RANK	STATEMENT	A %	GT %	PT %	GS %	PS %
20.	Experiential learning methods can feel unrealistic.	60	64	89	53	69

Key : A = All respondents (n=397)
    GT = General nurse tutors (n=109)
    PT = Psychiatric nurse tutors (n=26)
    GS = General nurse students (n=222)
    PS = Psychiatric nurse students (n=40)

Category 5 The General Tutors View

Nature of the Category : The statements in this category were items that represented the general tutors' viewpoint.

Criterion for Inclusion : Responses where there was a higher level of agreement to a statement by general nurse tutors than by any of the other groups and where there was an at least 5% higher rating by the general tutors than the next nearest category of respondents.

EXAMPLE

RANK	STATEMENT	A %	GT %	PT %	GS %	PS %
19.	Experiential learning can be a form of therapy for students.	62	74	65	55	68

Key : A = All respondents (n=397)
    GT = General nurse tutors (n=109)
    PT = Psychiatric nurse tutors (n=26)
    GS = General nurse students (n=222)
    PS = Psychiatric nurse students (n=40)

Category 6 The Psychiatric Students View

Nature of the Category : The statements in this category represented the psychiatric students' viewpoint.

Criteria for Inclusion : Responses where there was a higher level of agreement to a statement by psychiatric students than by any of the other groups and where there was an at least 5% higher rating by the psychiatric nursing students than the next nearest category of respondents.

EXAMPLE

RANK	STATEMENT	A %	GT %	PT %	GS %	PS %
17.5	Experiential learning is difficult to define.	64	61	50	66	72

Key : A = All respondents (n=397)
    GT = General nurse tutors (n=109)
    PT = Psychiatric nurse tutors (n=26)
    GS = General nurse students (n=222)
    PS = Psychiatric nurse students (n=40)

Category 7 The General Students View

Nature of the Category : The statements in this category represented the general students' viewpoint.

Criteria for Inclusion : Responses where there was a higher level of agreement to a statement by general students than by any of the other groups and where there was an at least 5% higher rating by the general nursing students than the next nearest category of respondents.

EXAMPLE

RANK	STATEMENT	A %	GT %	PT %	GS %	PS %
17.5	Experiential learning is 'practical' rather than 'theoretical' learning.	64	36	50	80	59

Key : A = All respondents (n=397)
     GT = General nurse tutors (n=109)
     PT = Psychiatric nurse tutors (n=26)
     GS = General nurse students (n=222)
     PS = Psychiatric nurse students (n=40)

Category 8 The Psychiatric Nurses' View

Nature of the Category : The statements in this category represented the psychiatric nurses' viewpoint (both tutors and students).
Criteria for Inclusion : Responses where there was a higher level of agreement between psychiatric nurse tutors and psychiatric nursing students than other groups.

EXAMPLE

RANK	STATEMENT	A %	GT %	PT %	GS %	PS %
10.5	School learning and clinical learning are not always linked.	78	84	92	72	92

Key : A = All respondents (n=397)
     GT = General nurse tutors (n=109)
     PT = Psychiatric nurse tutors (n=26)
     GS = General nurse students (n=222)
     PS = Psychiatric nurse students (n=40)

Category 9 The General Nurses' View

Nature of the Category : The statements in this category represented the general nurses' viewpoint (both tutors and students).
Criterion for Inclusion : Responses where there was a higher level of agreement between general nurse tutors and general nursing students than other groups.

EXAMPLE

RANK	STATEMENT	A %	GT %	PT %	GS %	PS %
15.	Experiential learning is not "textbook" learning.	69	72	65	69	62

Key : A = All respondents (n=397)
      GT = General nurse tutors (n=109)
      PT = Psychiatric nurse tutors (n=26)
      GS = General nurse students (n=222)
      PS = Psychiatric nurse students (n=40)

Category 10   Miscellaneous

Nature of the Category : The statements in this category were those that did not fall into any of the above.
Criterion for Inclusion : Responses that did not fit into any of the above categories.

The findings from this method of analysing the questionnaire data are identified in the next chapter.

9 Findings from the experiential learning survey

This chapter offers the findings from the questionnaire survey. It is divided into the following four sections :

- Characteristics of the respondents,
- Experiential learning methods,
- Perceptions of Experiential learning,
- Summary.

Characteristics of the Respondents

The overal response rate for the questionnaire was 77.9% or a total of 397 returned and completed questionnaires. The distribution of those responses can be seen in Table 9.1. In reading the findings below, it is important to bear in mind the differences in total numbers of respondents in each group. For the purposes of comparisons, percentages of responses are identified and discussed. Actual numbers of responses are indicated in square brackets.

Table 9.1
Return of Questionnaires

	Number Distributed	Number Returned	Response Rate %
General Tutors	150	109	72.6
Psychiatric Tutors	34	26	76.4
General Students	268	222	82.8
Psychiatric Students	57	40	70.1
Totals	509	397	77.9

In line with national trends in nursing, the majority of the respondent group were female. Most of the students were under the age of 30 (84% [186] of the general students and 65% [26] of the psychiatric students. Most of the tutors were over 31 (100% [26] of the psychiatric tutors and 90% [98] of the general tutors). This suggests a difference of at least one generation between most students and most tutors.

Experiential Learning Methods

The first part of the questionnaire asked respondents to identify the experiential learning methods they had either used or taken part in. All of the respondents had used or taken part in some experiential learning methods. More than 90% of the total sample [n = 397] had taken part in one or more of the following :
- small group activities (98%) [389]
- role play (96%) [381]
- practising clinical skills (94%) [373]
- icebreakers (92%) [365]

Analysis, by type of respondent demonstrated that more psychiatric tutors and students took part in those experiential learning methods lower down the scale. Psychiatric nursing students more

187

frequently acknowledged that they had taken part in reflective activities, simulations, empathy exercises and transactional analysis exercises than did general nursing students. Psychiatric nurse tutors more frequently stated that they had used or taken part in reflection, simulations, empathy exercises, transactional analysis exercises, gestalt exercises and psychodrama than did general nursing tutors. All psychiatric nurse tutors claimed that they had used or taken part in role play and icebreaker activities.

Overall, psychiatric nurses took part or were using more experiential learning methods than were general nurses with the exception of small group discussions, where general nurses reported a slightly higher response than psychiatric nurses. Table 9.6 illustrates the distribution of responses to the experiential learning methods questions. Frequency counts were undertaken for **all** the respondents' responses and a rank order list was produced from that computation. Then, frequency counts for each item, by type of respondent were identified and these are shown in the appropriate columns in Table 9.2.

Table 9.2
Rank Order : Identified Experiential Learning
Methods, by Percentage

RANK	EXPERIENTIAL LEARNING METHODS	LI%	GS%	PS%	PT%	GT%
1.	Small group discussion	98% 389	98% 218	98% 39	96% 25	98% 107
2.	Role Play	96% 382	96% 213	97% 38	100% 26	95% 104
3.	Practising Clinical Nursing Skills	94% 373	96% 213	87% 35	85% 22	95% 104
4.	Icebreaker activities	92% 365	87% 193	97% 38	100% 26	97% 106
5.	Structured group activities	84% 333	84% 186	85% 34	92% 24	84% 12
6.	Problem solving activities	83% 329	82% 182	83% 33	85% 22	87% 95
7.	Exercises that involve reflection on past or present experience	74% 294	67% 149	90% 36	86% 23	81% 88
8.	The "blind walk" exercise	72% 286	72% 160	74% 30	73% 19	70% 76
9.	Simulations	51% 202	43% 95	51% 20	86% 22	59% 64
10.	Empathy building exercises	47% 187	40% 89	62% 25	77% 20	50% 54

11.	Psychodrama	19%	18%	18%	39%	16%
		75	40	7	10	17
12.	Transactional	18%	11%	51%	46%	14%
	Analysis	71	24	20	12	15
	exercises					
13.	Gestalt	12%	11%	10%	19%	11%
	exercises	48	24	4	5	12

KEY :

ALL = All respondents (n = 397)
GS = General nursing students (n = 222)
PS = Psychiatric nursing students (n = 40)
PT = Psychiatric tutors (n = 26)
GT = General tutors (n = 109)

Uppper figures are percentages
Lower figures are numbers of respondents

Other Experiential Learning Activities Identified

Respondents were also invited to identify other learning activities that they considered to be "experiential". Of the total group, 39 identified other activities. More psychiatric nurse tutors identified "other" experiential learning methods than any other group of respondents (35% of the psychiatric tutor group).

The various activities identified by the respondents were grouped together under the following headings :

- clinical activities,
- classroom activities,
- use of technology
- self-awareness and therapy activities

The activities, classified in this way, are listed in appendix 4. What was notable about these "other" experiential learning methods was the breadth that they covered. It seemed as though, for some tutors, almost **any** teaching or learning activity could be described as experiential, with the exception of the lecture method.

Perceptions of Experiential Learning

As noted in the previous chapter, a method was devised for classifying responses to the Likert-type questions. The findings in each of those groupings will now be identified.

Category 1 : The Overall View of Experiential Learning in Nurse Education

A High Level of Agreement with Statements

It will be recalled that statements included in this section were those where there was a high level of agreement (above 82%) with statements, by all respondents in both student groups and both tutor groups. The statements can therefore be taken to represent the views of the whole group.

The statements in this section were :

- Experiential learning can be fun (92% agreement overall [365])
- Student nurses learn best from personal experience (91% agreement overall [361])
- Experiential learning is learning by doing (89% agreement overall [353]),
- Experiential learning methods encourage you to reflect on your nursing practice (88% agreement overall [349]),
- Experiential learning methods can increase self-awareness (88% agreement overall [349]),
- Experiential learning methods are useful for learning interpersonal skills (86% agreement overall [341]).

B. Low Level of Agreement with Statements

This section notes responses where tutors and students of all groups were in accord regarding agreement with a statement at a low level

191

(single figure percentages). In other words, these were the statements that were **most strongly disagreed with.**

The statements in this section were :

- I don't like experiential learning methods (8% agreement overall [32]),
- Experiential learning methods suit all teachers (4% agreement overall [16]).

Category 2 : The Tutors' View of Experiential Learning

Statements included in this section were those where there was there was a higher level of agreement to a statement in both tutor groups when compared to both student groups. The statements can therefore be taken to represent all of the tutors.

The statements in this section were :

- Experiential learning methods do not suit all students (85% agreement by general tutors [93] and 85% agreement by psychiatric tutors [22]),
- Experiential learning methods can be time consuming (80% agreement by general tutors [87] and 81% agreement by psychiatric tutors [21]).
- Experiential learning methods can be embarrassing (89% agreement by psychiatric nurse tutors [23] and 83% agreement by general tutors [90]).

There were considerable differences in response to the second item, above, between the tutor and student groups. Only 66% [26] of the psychiatric nursing student group agreed with the statement regarding experiential learning methods being time consuming and only 56% [118] of the general nursing students .

The statement concerning embarrassment was also agreed with by a high percentage of psychiatric nursing students and psychiatric nursing tutors and is discussed under the "miscellaneous" category, below. The statement is also included in the psychiatric nurses category.

192

Category 3 : The Students' Views of Experiential Learning

Statements included in this section where those where there was a higher level of agreement to a statement in both student groups when compared to both student groups. The statements can therefore be taken to represent all of the students.

The statements in this section were :

- Experiential learning methods are easy to take part in (53% agreement by general students [118] and 44% agreement by psychiatric students [18]).
- Experiential learning methods are easier to use than other learning methods (38% agreement by general students [84] and 33% agreement by psychiatric students [13])

In this section, slightly more than half of the general student group agreed that experiential learning methods were easy to take part in and slightly less than half of the psychiatric students agreed. On the other hand, only 38% [84] of the general students and 33% [13] of the psychiatric students agreed that they were easier to take part in than other methods, indicating that **more** students disagreed with this statement than agreed with it. Thus it can be said that, on the whole, the students did NOT feel that experiential learning methods are easier to use than other learning methods. In the other groups, only 21% [23] of the general tutors agreed with this statement and only 8% [3] of the psychiatric nurse tutors agreed that experiential learning methods were easier to use than other methods.

Category 4 : The Psychiatric Tutors' Views of Experiential Learning

Statements included in this section were those where there was a higher level of agreement to a statement by psychiatric nurse tutors than by any of the other groups and where there was an at least 5% higher rating by the psychiatric tutors than the next nearest category of respondents. The statements can therefore be taken to represent the views of the psychiatric nurse tutors.

The statements in this section were :

- Experiential learning methods can feel unrealistic (89% of psychiatric tutors [23]),
- Experiential learning is concerned with learning more about how you feel (73% of psychiatric tutors [19]),
- Experiential learning is learning that takes place in the clinical setting (73% of psychiatric tutors [29]),
- Experiential learning sessions could get out of control (85% of psychiatric tutors [22]),
- Experiential learning can be a form of therapy for tutors (62% of psychiatric tutors [16]),
- I prefer experiential learning methods to other learning methods (60% of psychiatric tutors [16])

The psychiatric nurse tutors were well ahead in their percentage agreement to two of these statements. Whilst 89% [23] of them felt that experiential learning methods can feel unrealistic, only 69% [28] of the psychiatric students did, 64% [70] of the general tutors did and only 53% [118] of the general nursing students did. On the issue of experiential learning methods having potential for getting out of control, 85% [22] of the psychiatric tutors agreed with this statement, whilst 77% [84] of the general tutors did. The students had lower percentage ratings to this item : 56% [22] of the psychiatric students agreed with the statement, whilst only 44% [98] of the general students did.

On the issue of preferring experiential learning methods to other learning methods, the psychiatric nurse tutors were again ahead by a considerable degree. In all of the other cases, less than 50% agreed with the statement, indicating that **only** psychiatric nurse tutors preferred the methods to other methods (39% [16] psychiatric nursing students, 34% [37] general tutors, 34% [75] general nursing students).

Category 5 : The General Nurse Tutors' View of Experiential Learning

Statements included in this section were those where there was a higher level of agreement to a statement by general nurse tutors than by any of the other groups and where there was an at least 5% higher rating by the general tutors than the next nearest category of respondents. The statements can therefore be taken to represent the views of the general nurse tutors.

The statements in this section were :

- Experiential learning can be a form of therapy for students (74% of general tutors [81]),
- Experiential learning does not involve lectures (47% of general tutors [51]).
- Experiential learning methods can be embarrassing (83% of general tutors [90]).

It may be noted, here, that less than half of the general tutors agreed that "experiential learning does not involve lectures. This may be compared to the other groups, where 23% [6] of the psychiatric tutors agreed with the statement, 24% [53] of the general students and 18% [7] of the psychiatric students. It may therefore be concluded that most of the respondent did not agree that experiential learning does not involve lectures.

The issue of embarrassment was also agreed with by high percentages of psychiatric nursing tutors and psychiatric nursing students and is included in the "psychiatric nursing" category, below, and discussed in the "miscellaneous" category, below.

Category 6 : The Psychiatric Nursing Students' View of Experiential Learning

Statements included in this section were those where there was a higher level of agreement to a statement by psychiatric students than by any of the other groups and where there was an at least 5% higher rating by the psychiatric nursing students than the next nearest category of respondents. The statements can therefore be taken to represent the views of psychiatric nursing students.

The statements in this section were :

- Experiential learning method used in the school are useful for learning about nursing (90% of psychiatric students [36])
- Experiential learning methods help students to learn practical nursing skills (90% of psychiatric students [36]).

195

- Experiential learning is difficult to define (72% of psychiatric students [29]),
- Student nurses are allowed to negotiate their learning programmes with their tutors (85% of psychiatric students [34]),
- Experiential learning methods are the best methods for learning about nursing (49% of psychiatric students [19]),
- Students are free to choose the learning methods that suit them best (54% of psychiatric students [22]),
- Student nurses learn most about nursing in the school of nursing (21 % of psychiatric students [8]).

Whilst psychiatric students clearly thought that experiential learning methods helped them to learn about nursing and to learn practical nursing skills, less that half felt that they were the **best** methods of learning about nursing. Psychiatric nursing students had different views about the **nature** of their educational experience than did general students. 85% [34] of the psychiatric nursing students felt that they were allowed to negotiate their learning programmes with their tutors, whilst only 77% [171] of the general students felt they could. Also, 54% [22] of the psychiatric students felt that they were free to choose the learning method that suits them best, whilst only 27% [60] of the general students felt that **they** were.

Whilst only a small percentage of psychiatric nurses agreed that student nurses learn most about nursing in the school of nursing (21% [8]), thus indicating that a larger proportion **disagreed with** or were uncertain about the statement, it is notable that very much smaller percentages of people in other groups agreed with the statement : **no** psychiatric nurse tutors agree with it, 3% [3] of general nurse tutors agreed with it and 4% [9] of general nursing students agreed with it.

Category 7 : The General Nursing Students' View of Experiential Learning

Statements included in this section were those where there was a higher level of agreement to a statement by general students than by any of the other groups and where there was an at least 5% higher rating by the general nursing students than the next nearest category of respondents. The statements can therefore be taken as representing the views of the general nursing students.

The statements in this section were :

- Students learn most about nursing in the clinical situation (90% of general students [200]).
- Experiential learning is "practical" learning rather than 'theoretical' learning (80% of general students [178]).

Only 54% of the psychiatric nursing students agreed with the statement that " students learn most about nursing in the clinical situation. Also, only 59% [24] of psychiatric nursing students agreed with the statement that "experiential learning is "practical" learning rather than "theoretical" learning and only 36% [39] of the general tutors and 50% [13] of the psychiatric nurse tutors agreed with the statement.

Category 8 : The Psychiatric Nurses' View of Experiential Learning

Statements included in this section were those where there was a higher level of agreement between psychiatric nurse tutors and psychiatric nursing students than other groups. The statements can therefore be taken as representing the overall views of the psychiatric nurses in the sample.

The statements in this section were :

- "School" learning and "clinical" learning are not always linked (92% of the psychiatric tutors [24] and 92% of the psychiatric nursing students [37]),
- Experiential learning methods can be used in the clinical setting (92% of the psychiatric tutors [24] and 90% of the psychiatric nursing students [36]).
- Experiential learning is learning from life experience (87% of the psychiatric nursing students [35] and 85% of the psychiatric tutors [22]).
- Experiential learning methods can be embarrassing (89% of the psychiatric nursing tutors [23] and 85% of the psychiatric nursing students [34].)

Notable, in both these instances, was the degree of agreement between the psychiatric nurses when compared to the general nurses.

For the "school" and "clinical" question, 84% [91] of the general tutors and 72% [160] of the general students agreed with the statement. For the "clinical settings" question, 74% [81] of the general tutors and 70% [155] of the general students agreed with the statement.

With regard to the issue of experiential learning being learning from life experience, the general nurse tutors were close behind the psychiatric nurse tutors with 83% [90] agreement with the statement. Fewer of the general nursing students agreed with the statement (67% [149]).

The issue of embarrassment was highly endorsed by general tutors as well as by psychiatric nurses and is included in the general nurse tutors category and is also discussed in the "miscellaneous" category, below.

Category 9 : The General Nurses' View of Experiential Learning

Statements included in this section were those where there was a higher level of agreement between general nurse tutors and general nursing students than other groups. The statements can therefore be taken as representing the overall views of the general nurses in the sample.

The statements in this section were :

• Experiential learning is not "textbook" learning (72% of the general tutors [78] and 69% of the general nursing students [153]).

• Students learn most about nursing by observing other nurses at work (56% of the general nursing students [124] and 51% of the general tutors [55]).

Whilst more than half of the general nurses agreed that students learn most about nursing by observing other nurses at work, fewer than half of the psychiatric nursing groups did (42% [11] of the psychiatric nurse tutors and 36% [14] of the psychiatric nursing students).

Category 10 : Miscellaneous

Statements included in this section were those that did not fit easily into any other category.

The statements in this section were :

- Experiential learning methods can be embarrassing,
- Experiential learning methods are suitable for learning all aspects of nursing.

Here, responses were mixed and are illustrated in Table 9.8

Table 9.8
Responses to Two Statements

STATEMENT	ALL	GT	PT	GS	PS
Experiential learning methods can be embarrassing	77% [306]	83% [90]	89% [23]	71% [158]	85% [34]
Experiential learning methods are suitable for learning all aspects of nursing.	19% [75]	10% [11]	27% [7]	23% [51]	10% [4]

KEY :

ALL = All respondents (n = 397)
GT = General tutors (n = 109)
PT = Psychiatric tutors (n = 26)
GS = General students (n = 222)
PS = Psychiatric students (n = 40)

Whilst there was a generally high level of agreement to the statement that "experiential learning can be embarrassing", the percentage of agreement was highest amongst the psychiatric nurse tutors and psychiatric nursing students, closely followed by the general nurse tutors. Given these high percentage figures, this statement was included in the nurse tutor and psychiatric nursing student categories. There was generally a low level of agreement with the statement about experiential learning methods being suitable for learning all aspects of nursing but there was a slightly higher level of agreement to it in the psychiatric nurse tutors and general nursing students groups. On the whole, though, it can be seen that more people **disagreed** with or were uncertain about the statement than agreed with it, across all groups.

Summary

In the presentation of findings, above, all of the questionnaire responses were accounted for. All of the perceptions identified above are brought together, below, in a summary of the perceptions of the various groups.

All of the respondents had taken part in some experiential learning activities. The activities most frequently used or taken part in were small group activities, role play, practising clinical skills and icebreakers. The psychiatric nursing respondents had a broader experience of experiential learning activities and tended to have taken part in or used more of the "humanistic" or therapy-based approaches than had the general nursing respondents.

Turning to the respondents perceptions of experiential learning, the picture that emerged from **most** of the respondents includes the following characteristics. Experiential learning was fun, it was learning by doing, involved reflection and it was generally popular. It could be used to teach interpersonal skills and could enhance self-awareness. It was generally felt, too, that students learn best from personal experience. Most respondents felt that experiential learning methods did not suit all teachers.

From the tutors point of view, experiential learning could be time consuming and did not suit all learners. On the other hand, the students generally felt that experiential learning methods were easy to take part in, if embarrasing at times.

The psychiatric nurse tutors emphasised the affective aspects of experiential learning, felt that experiential learning sessions could get out of control and that they could be a form of therapy for tutorial staff. They tended to prefer experiential learning methods to other learning and teaching methods although felt that such methods could be unrealistic.

The general tutors felt that experiential learning methods could be a form of therapy for students and that experiential learning did not usually involve lectures.

Whilst the psychiatric nursing students sometimes felt that experiential learning could be difficult to define, they often felt that they were a useful way of learning about nursing skills. They also tended to state that they could negotiated their learning programmes and were free to choose the learning methods that suited them best. A higher percentage of psychiatric nursing students than any other group felt that they learned most about nursing in the school or nursing. On the other hand, the general nursing students emphasised that they learned most about nursing in the clinical setting and stressed that experiential learning was "practical" rather than "theoretical" learning.

The psychiatric nurses, as a group, felt that school and clinical work were not always linked, that experiential learning was often learning from life experience and that experiential learning methods could be embarrasing. They also felt that experiential learning methods could be used in the clinical setting. The general nurses, as a group, felt that experiential learning was different to "textbook" learning and that students learn most about nursing by observing other nurses at work.

What was noticeable was that the psychiatric nurses of both tutor and student groups had a greater diversity of strongly held views than did the general nursing groups.

10 Experiential learning: Comparisons and contrasts

In this chapter, the similarities and differences between the findings from the interviews and the findings from the questionnaire are compared and contrasted. In the final chapter, the themes from this one will be explored in more detail.

Experiential Learning Methods

Both the interviews and the questionnaire identified that a wide range of experiential learning methods were used, although more and a wider range were used in psychiatric nursing than in general nursing. The experiential learning method that was most frequently cited was that of role play and this was also the one that came in for a lot of criticism from students during their interviews. It was role play that tended to prompt the cry of "embarrassing" from the students.

Common Themes : Interviews and Questionnaire

In this section, the particular characteristics that were constant themes throughout the interview and questionnaire data are presented. Three headings have been developed :

- Shared tutor and student perceptions of experiential learning. These perceptions are ones that were found in both the interviews and the questionnaire responses of both tutors and students.
- Tutor perceptions of experiential learning. These perceptions are ones that were found in both the interviews and the questionnaires of the tutors.
- Student perceptions of experiential learning. These perceptions are ones that were found in both the interviews and the questionnaires of the students,

The Characteristics of Experiential Learning as Perceived by both Tutors and Students Through Interview and Questionnaire

Key issues emerged from both the interviews and the questionnaires that could be said to represent the views of both samples of tutors and students through both the interviews and the questionnaire. They can be divided up into two groups : characteristics of experiential learning and experiential learning methods.

Experiential learning

Experiential learning can be fun.
Experiential learning is personal learning.
Experiential learning is learning by doing.
Experiential learning involves reflection.
Experiential learning can increase self-awareness
Experiential learning can help in the development of interpersonal skills.

In summary, here, it is noticeable that experiential learning was characterised as an **active** and **personal** approach to learning. It involved reflection on what was happening and (possibly as a result of that reflection) it tended to increase self-awareness, although it should be recalled that, when challenged, the tutors being interviewed found it difficult to define exactly what they meant by the term "self-awareness". Notable, too, was the fact that experiential learning was "fun" - not a descriptor that is commonly used in conjunction with educational activities. Indeed Henry (1989) in her study of 52 educators' perceptions of experiential learning expressed surprise that "virtually no on volunteered fun or enjoyment as an outcome"(Henry 1989 p35).

Experiential learning methods

The terms "experiential learning" and "experiential learning methods were sometimes used as synonyms and sometimes used to describe a) and approach to learning (experiential learning) and b) a type of learning activity (experiential learning methods). The comments from the interviews and questionnaire that referred explicitly to **experiential learning methods** were negative in nature and were as follows :

Experiential learning methods can be embarrassing.
Experiential learning methods can be unreal.
Experiential learning methods don"t suit all learners.

It is interesting to note that despite experiential learning being "fun", it could also be embarrassing, perhaps suggesting that a degree of embarrassment can also be enjoyable. The issue of unrealness was often noted in conjunction with experiential learning methods used in the school of nursing. This underlines a trend towards the students perceiving experiential learning as being more to do with learning in the clinical setting and to do with learning by observing other nurses at work. It seemed that the setting up of activities in the school of nursing often led to a pale imitation of the "real thing". It was noted, too, that experiential learning methods did not always suit all learners. In the student interviews, this was often linked to role play as an activity. A number of students felt that either a) role play did not suit some of their colleagues or b) role play did not suit them.
In summary, it appears that when experiential learning is viewed overall, as a learning strategy that involves learning from personal experience and learning by doing, the process is enjoyable.

However, the use of particular activities that can be called "experiential learning methods" may lead to embarrassment and a sense of unreality.

The Characteristics of Experiential Learning as Perceived by TUTORS Through Interview and Questionnaire

Tutors seemed to focus on the **practical** and procedural aspects of experiential learning. The characteristics that they identified were:

Experiential learning is concerned with feelings.
Experiential learning methods are not suitable for teaching or learning all topics on the syllabus.
Experiential learning methods could get out of control.
Experiential learning can be time consuming.

All but the first of these characteristics is to do with the organisation of learning activities and processes. Given the concern about experiential learning methods getting out of control, even the first item ("experiential learning is concerned with feelings") may also be an organisational issue. It seems possible that a number of tutors were worried about what might happen if experiential learning methods led to students becoming emotionally distressed. This issue was frequently discussed in the interviews.

The fact that a large percentage of tutors felt that experiential learning could be both time consuming and could get out of control suggests that tutors may prefer to maintain control over the **structure** of a student's learning experience. This is further borne out by the idea that experiential learning methods are not suitable for teaching or learning all topics on the syllabus, although it should be noted that such a sentiment was not a **universal** one amongst the tutors. In interview, at least one tutor felt that **everything** could be taught experientially. Some tutors were particularly "sold" on the experiential learning approach and one commented that it was his favourite approach to learning and teaching.

The Characteristics of Experiential Learning as Perceived by STUDENTS Through Interview and Questionnaire

The students tended to see experiential learning as being concerned with the clinical setting. When they **did** refer to experiential learning in the school of nursing, the accent was on learning "practical skills" rather than on "academic" issues. They noted, too, that school and clinical learning where not always linked. The characteristics identified here were :

Experiential learning is "practical" rather than "theoretical" learning.
Experiential learning is clinical learning.
"School" learning and "clinical" learning are not always linked.

Psychiatric and General Nursing

Differences were found between the ways in which psychiatric nurses and general nurses perceived experiential learning. These differences could only be found through analysis of the questionnaire responses as the interview data was not divided up according to nursing discipline. On the other hand, it should be borne in mind that the questionnaire was developed out of the interview data and thus reflects the perceptions of the interviewees.

The Characteristics of Experiential Learning In Psychiatric Nursing:

a. Tutors Perceptions
Experiential learning is concerned with feelings.
Experiential learning could get out of control.
Experiential learning can be therapy for the tutors.

b. Students Perceptions
Experiential learning methods are useful for learning about nursing.
Experiential learning methods help students to learn practical nursing skills.
Students are allowed to negotiate their own learning programmes.
Students are free to choose their own learning methods.

First, the accent in the psychiatric nurses picture of experiential learning is that there is an emphasis on the "feelings" and "therapy" aspects of experiential learning. It should be noted, too, that the psychiatric nurses were more familiar with the "humanistic" types of experiential learning methods such as psychodrama and transactional analysis activities : all of which had developed out of a **therapeutic** context, as discussed in the first chapter.

Second, the students in psychiatric nurses **liked** experiential learning methods and found them useful for learning about nursing. Also, they acknowledged that they were more free to negotiate their own learning programmes than was the case for general students and felt that they were free to choose their own learning methods. In the end, of course, **everyone** is free to choose his or her own learning method as presumably we **only** learn through our own particular method. The students' perception of learning, though, seems to suggest that they feel they are engaged in a more democratic learning process than the general students.

The Characteristics of Experiential Learning in General Nursing :

a. Tutors Perceptions
Experiential learning can be therapy for the students
Experiential learning methods can be embarrassing.
b. Students Perceptions
Students learn most about nursing in the clinical setting
Experiential learning is "practical" rather than "theoretical" learning.

It was more difficult to filter out **particular** characteristics of experiential learning for general nurses. The tutors felt that experiential learning could be therapy for students and felt that experiential learning methods could be embarrassing. For the students, the accent was on **practical** learning and on the clinical setting rather than on the school of nursing. As noted, above, the general nurses had less experience of the more "therapeutic" or humanistic types of experiential learning methods, when compared to the psychiatric nurses.

Given that the psychiatric nursing group, from the questionnaire point of view, was a smaller group, it is interesting to note that the psychiatric nurses generally had more to say about experiential learning than did the general nurses. It was noted, earlier, that the

207

1982 syllabus of training for psychiatric nurses had **prescribed** the use of experiential learning methods and from the results obtained here, it is evident that, in Wales at least, more experiential learning methods are being used in psychiatric nurse training than are being used in general nurse training. Also, the psychiatric nurses tended to see experiential learning methods used in the school of nursing as more relevant to the process of becoming a nurse than did the students in general training, who tended to identify **clinical work** as being of most relevance.

11 A review of the experiential learning study

This evaluative chapter reviews aspects of the study relating to methodology, validity, analysis and limitations. It leads to the final chapter which offers a detailed discussion of the overall findings. Many of the issues in this chapter have been referred to at points throughout this report. The aim, here, is to bring them together.

Aims of the Study

The stated aim of the study was to explore nurse tutors' and student nurses' perceptions of experiential learning. This aim was achieved through a two pronged approach : first, through in-depth interviews with tutors and students and then through a survey in which a questionnaire was used that was developed out of the interview data. The questionnaire survey was limited to the principality of Wales in order to enable a total population of tutors to be survey.

Methods

Initially, interviews were conducted with 12 tutors from various parts of the UK and 12 students who had been taught by some of those tutors. These two groups provided a wealth of information that was analysed by two methods : a simple content analysis of themes and a more detailed qualitative analysis in the style of grounded theory. The numbers in these two samples proved sufficient to allow for themes to begin to be repeated by the respondents. By the 9th interview with the tutors and by the 7th interview with the students, the same sorts of themes and ideas were being expressed again and again thus theoretical sampling can be said to have been satisfactory.

The questionnaire was developed directly out of the findings from the two sets of interviews. Face validity was established through the use of a panel of experts and the researcher asked one of the interviewees to review the questionnaire as well. The aim, here, was to explore the degree to which those themes discussed in the interviews were supported (or not supported) by a wider range of tutors and students. One omission in the questionnaire was reference to the theme raised by a number of tutors : that experiential learning could be uncomfortable or threatening to students. In retrospect, it is difficult to account for why this was left out and it would be included in any further survey of this sort.

The reasonably good response rate (for a postal questionnaire) of 77.9% and the prompt return of the questionnaires suggest that they were relatively easy to fill in and/or administer. It is felt that personal contact with the senior tutors responsible for distributing the questionnaires in various parts of Wales helped to ensure speedy completion.

The processing of the data produced from the questionnaire was labour intensive and time consuming. In future studies, a separate column for coding each of the questionnaire items would be incorporated into the questionnaire design.

Validity and Reliability

Validity and reliability are important aspects of all research and is particularly vital in qualitative work where the researcher's subjectivity can so readily cloud the interpretation of the data.

Various elements of validity and reliability checking were built into each stage of this project.

Following each initial category generation during the content analyses of the interviews, two people who had nothing to do with the project were invited to generate **their own** category systems. These were then compared to the researcher's system and a final category system was negotiated through discussion. This allowed for both reliability **and** validity checks. The method checked **reliability** of the system by ensuring that the researcher and two other people were consistently generating similar category systems. It checked for **validity** in that it attempted to ensure that the category systems really reflected the content of the interview transcripts. Further checks for validity were carried out, later, by returning to a number of respondents to ask them to review the analyses for the degree to which they reflected the respondents' perceptions. A "common sense" rule had to apply here. It was impossible to ask every respondent to check the analyses. Thus, once three respondents had found the analyses satisfactory, it was accepted by the researcher that it was likely that he had represented the other respondent's views fairly.

When the questionnaire was developed, a "panel of experts" was invited to review the questionnaire. Again, elements of both reliability and face validity checking were present here. The panel checked for validity by helping to ensure that the questionnaire reasonably reflected the findings from the interview data. The panel checked for reliability by attempting to identify ambiguous questions. One measure of a reliable questionnaire would be that each item in it would be understood by each respondent in the same way.

The questionnaire had been developed from the words and phrases used by the interviewees in the first stage of the research project. The literature on experiential learning had also been consulted prior to constructing the questionnaire. These two factors helped to enhance content validity (Nieswieadomy 1987). The validity of the questionnaire was further established by discussing it with one of the interview respondents to ensure that it reflected the things that interviewees had discussed. Again, this helped to enhance both face and content validity. Nieswieadomy (1987) notes that :

> The actual degree of content validity is never established; an instrument possesses some degree of validity that can only be estimated. (Nieswieadomy 1987 : 102).

The issue of establishing validity in qualitative research and in the theory that is generated from it is also problematic. Degerando, an explorer, writing in 1800 summarised some of the problems well :

The first fault that we notice in the observations on savages is their incompleteness; it was only to be expected, given the shortness of their stay, the division of their attention, and the absence of any regular tabulation of their findings. (Degerando 1800 [1969] : 65).

Whilst, in this study, the tabulation of findings was carried out satisfactorily, the problem of whether or not the interviews were long enough and whether or not attention was always focussed on the "right" issues, remain problematic. On the other hand, Webb et al (1966) suggest that one of the most successful ways of addressing the validity issue is through the use of multiple methods. It is asserted, here, that the use of interviews and questionnaires and reference back to the literature helped in the search for validity.

Questionnaire Analysis

The analyses of the interviews have been discussed in detail earlier in this report. Chapter 8 also described how the questionnaire data were analysed. The point needs reinforcing, here, that no attempt was made to use detailed statistical methods of analyses. First, the tutor sample was a **total** one and thus findings from the questionnaires would always reflect the perceptions of the tutor respondents and, in turn, be representative of the perceptions of a large proportion of all of the tutors in Wales. Second, the individual samples (general tutors, psychiatric tutors, general students, psychiatric students) varied in size. Also, the student samples were not randomly selected. The type of data produced by a large section of the questionnaire was **ordinal**. Finally, no hypotheses were being tested in this study. Following advice from two statisticians, therefore, it was decided to limit the analysis to frequency counts and a comparison of percentages of responses in order to offer a descriptive picture of tutors' and students' perceptions of experiential learning. No attempt was being made to generalise the findings from this study.

A Specific Limitation

An interesting limitation that has not been discussed so far is a slightly complicated and puzzling one. It is that there were perceived differences between the data emerging from interviews **as those interviews happened** and the data that were found in the written transcripts. Often, the interview seemed to be clear and full of detailed information. The transcripts, on the other hand, although they contained the words spoken by the interviewees often seemed more difficult to "understand". Thus, what seemed to have been an exiting, thought-provoking and clear interview was somehow transformed into something far more prosaic when transferred to paper. The researcher has discussed this issue with a number of other researchers who have reported similar findings. There seems to be a need for a method of capturing the "indescribable something" of the live interview. Ironically, this illustrates the issue of the "experiential" philosophy precisely.

The closing chapter offers a detailed discussion of all of the findings of the study.

12 Clarifying the theory, learning the language and acquiring the values: The problem of the cultural isogloss

This chapter explores the findings of the study and attempts to identify how the various groups perceived experiential learning and the implications of those perceptions. It develops **two** levels of analysis. The first level of analysis is the one that most of the discussion has been concerned with so far : the explicit content of the interviews and questionnaires. The second level of analysis focuses only on the interviews and the literature. That analysis is concerned with certain "themes" that emerge out of the language being used by the interviewees and in the literature. This second level analysis is a more abstract form of analysis and is necessarily tentative.

First level analysis : analysis of explicit content of interviews and questionnaires. The methods used in this analysis were content analysis and a modified form of grounded theory. A phenomenological approach.

Second level analysis : analysis of apparent themes in the interviews and literature. The method used in this analysis involved looking at the language and ideas expressed in the interviews and literature to identify common styles of language and values. This level of analysis is more abstract and less concrete than the first level. It is necessarily more tentative and less easily validated than the previous level. An interpretative approach.

Terminology

Throughout this study, it became apparent that sometimes the terms "experiential learning" and "experiential learning methods" were used as synonyms and at other times they were used to denote a) an approach to learning (experiential learning) and b) a learning method or activity (experiential learning methods).

Experiential Learning Methods

When the question about "methods" was explicit (as, for example, it was in the questionnaire) and respondents were asked to identify experiential learning methods that they had used or taken part in, the response was that most had taken part in a range of methods. All had taken part in some experiential learning methods. From the questionnaire findings, it was clear that most had taken part in small group activities (98%), role play (96%) and activities that encouraged the practising of clinical skills (94%). As we noted in chapter 9, however, more psychiatric tutors and students had taken part in or used the more "humanistic" or "therapy oriented" methods such as psychodrama, transactional analysis exercises and gestalt exercises, although the numbers acknowledging their use of these was still small.

Again, as noted in chapter 9, questionnaire respondents were invited to list "other" experiential learning methods that they had used or taken part in. Those methods could be grouped together under the following four heads :

- Clinical activities,
- Classroom activities,
- Use of technology,
- Self-awareness and therapy activities.

This list seems to indicate that some respondents felt that most sorts of teaching activities (and some teaching "aids") could be classified as examples of experiential learning methods. For some, groups of activities were lumped together, as in "communications exercises" and "management training". On the whole, however, what is common to all of the above "methods" (apart, possibly, from lecturing) is that the learner is **active**. Thus the notion of experiential learning as "learning by doing" is further endorsed.

A number of "humanistic" activities were to be found here. Guided phantasy, for example, has been described in the humanistic and transpersonal literature on teaching and learning methods (Stevens 1971). Neurolinguistic programming is a particular approach to learning interactive skills, based on the work of Bandler and Grinder (1975, 1982). Bandler and Grinder studied three humanistic therapists at work and attempted to identify the behaviours that made those therapists "effective". They then began to teach those behaviours to others, working on the principle that other if others could learn the behaviours, they could become effective therapists.

Trust exercises have also been described in the humanistic literature (Kilty 1983, Heron 1982) and usually involve activities such as students falling backwards into one another's arms. The aim of such activities is to test out the degree to which we trust other people, with ourselves.

The "shop-mobility" exercise, in which students spend some part of the day in a city centre, in a wheelchair, in order to experience something of what it may be like to be handicapped is a variant of an similar activity described in the nursing press by Richardson, Bishop, Caygill et al (1990).

Overall, it can be stated that whilst all of the respondents had taken part in a selection of experiential learning methods, such methods were more frequently used in psychiatric nurse education than in general nurse education. This is hardly suprising, perhaps, given the 1982 syllabus of training for psychiatric nursing's prescription of such methods in psychiatric nurse training (ENB 1982). The point, though, is that a large number of educators and students in nursing are now using experiential learning methods.

The Overall Perceptions of Experiential Learning

As we noted in the previous chapter, certain characteristics of experiential learning were agreed by most respondents in both the

interviews and the questionnaire responses. These can be grouped together to answer four questions :
- What is experiential learning?
- What is it like?
- What is it useful for?
- What "type" of experiential learning are nurses involved in?

By developing answers to these four questions we can begin to identify various dimensions of perception on the part of the respondents in this study.

What is experiential learning?

The three statements that answer this question for the majority of respondents, both in the interviews and in the questionnaires are the following :
- It is learning by doing,
- It is personal learning,
- It involves reflection

Experiential learning, then, is an active rather than a passive form of learning. Often in the interviews, it was contrasted with "lecturing" or by "being taught". The idea of learning by doing suggests activity on the part of the learner and is in line with the Kolb (1984) view of experiential learning. The fact that it involves "doing", also suggests skills-learning (which is developed further in this chapter). To be engaged in "doing" something, suggests more that just thinking or puzzling, it suggests psychomotor activity.

Second, the suggestion is that experiential learning is personal learning : learning that makes a difference to the individual "personal" stock of knowledge. As we noted in the first chapter, Rogers (1967), Heron (1981) and Burnard (1987a) have all described "personal knowledge", following Polanyi's (1958) suggestion that we "know more than we can say". The suggestion, here, is that "personal knowledge" can be compared and contrasted with "public knowledge" or knowledge that is known by many other people. Again, this learning of personal knowledge links well with the idea of learning by doing and contrasts well with the lecture method of teaching and learning. The idea seems to be that in experiential learning, we learn by taking part and learn something that is personal to us, whereas in the lecture approach, we are more passive : we adopt knowledge from the "public

217

domain". This difference between the lecturer and experiential learning has been highlighted recently by Jones who suggested that :

Nursing as a whole appears to have grasped the concept of "experiential" learning with both hands, perhaps to the detriment of the lecture. (Jones 1990 : 290).

Finally, the characteristic of reflection was noted by most respondents. The suggestion, here, is that experiential learning involves not only **doing** something but that the person also **reflects** on what he or she is doing in order to learn. Figure 12.2 illustrates this process in action.

1. An Experience

2. Reflection on that experience

3. Development of Personal knowledge

Figure 12.2 An Experiential Learning Cycle Based on The Research Study

In this cycle, the person "does" something (has an experience), reflects on it and adds to his or her stock of personal knowledge. This cycle has much in common with Kolb's (1984) experiential learning cycle, discussed in chapter 1 although it suggests a **simplification** of his cycle. At least two points need to be made about such a cycle. First, there may be no guarantee that a person moves round the cycle. It would be quite possible, for instance, to have an experience, reflect on it and learn little as a result. We might, for example, just note what was happening to us and leave it at that. What the respondents in this study seem to suggest, however, is that experiential learning involves **all three** of the aspects of this cycle : doing, reflecting and personally learning.

The second point is that the cycle could, in theory, become a "closed loop". The individual could travel around it doing things, reflecting on his or her action and adding to his or her store of personal knowledge without changing his or her behaviour in the "real world". It would be hoped, however, that as the person works round the cycle, the "doing" aspect of it would involve using some of the personal learning from the previous stage to modify action or behaviour. Used in this way, it would be very like the problem solving cycle or the action learning cycle (Garrett 1983) in which a type of scientific process is undertaken by the individual. In this approach, something happens to the person, he or she reflects on what has happened, makes up "hypotheses" about what may happen next and acts accordingly. Depending on the outcome of his or her action, the person modifies that hypobook accordingly. This is the process that George Kelly described as the "man as scientist" (Kelly 1955). Kelly argued that this is how most of us live out our lives. We are constantly reflecting on what happens to us and predicting, as a result of that reflection, what will happen next. What we do next depends very much on that prediction. If our prediction proves correct, we carry on with our set of predictions. If it proves wrong, we "rewrite" our hypotheses.

The model of learning has much to commend it in nursing education. We noted, for example, that many of the students in this study saw experiential learning in terms of clinical learning. The cycle, above, could easily be made explicit to students as one to help them make sense of what happens to them in the clinical domain. The student who is able to reflect on what he or she does should be able to make constant adjustments to his or her stock of personal knowledge and, as a result, slightly modify his or her behaviour in the clinical setting as that becomes necessary. The key issue, here, seems to be **remembering to reflect**. The mystic, Ouspenksy (Reyner 1984) noted how easy it was to merely let life occur and to not notice what was happening to us. Reflection seems to call for a **conscious decision** to notice what is happening and to study what is happening. Mezirow noted that the process of being able to reflect is one of the features that marks us out as human (Mezeiro 1981). These aspects of reflection allow for the development of change – both change in the self (which will be addressed later in this chapter) and change in the situation (in this case, nursing). The nurse who can both reflect and develop critical awareness based on that reflection seems more likely to be able to live with and create change than one who merely reflects on and notices the status quo.

It was the students, in this study, who appeared to be more challenging of the status quo than were the tutors. This can be interpreted in at least two ways. First, it might suggest that the "new" system of education was "working" and that students were becoming more critical as a result of that system. Alternatively, it might be argued that tutors, for whatever reason, were becoming less critical as they pursued their careers. Later, it will be argued that the tutors and students in this study tended to occupy different "life worlds" : the students tended to "live" in the clinical setting, whilst the tutors tended to "live" in the school of nursing. Arguably, the school of nursing may be a more insular setting than the clinical one and a setting less likely to encourage a challenging of what is going on in the clinical setting.

The students in this study tended to take a pragmatic view of the educational system and were generally more concerned with the difference that system might make to them as **nurses.** The tutors tended to be rather more interested in the difference the educational system might make to students as **people.** A balance needs to be struck between a view of education and training which is purely instrumental (and thus set up only to produce effective nurses) and a view of education and training that has as it aim "personal growth". Neither views need be mutually exclusive nor should either view prevail at the expense of the other. The reflective process, then, is not just a reflection on "what does this mean in terms of me?" but also a reflection on "what does this mean for nursing?"

What is Experiential Learning like?

The next issue regards what experiential learning is like to take part in. The most frequently cited characteristics, here, were that it is **fun** and that it can be **embarrassing** (although it should be noted that the general nursing students in the study were less likely to see experiential learning as embarrassing than were the other groups. Even so, 72% of the general students in the questionnaire part of the study acknowledged that experiential learning could be embarrassing).

At first sight, these two characteristics seem to be almost contradictory. It might seem odd to view something as "fun and embarrassing". However, bearing in mind the characteristics of experiential learning described above : doing, reflecting and modifying personal experience, it seems possible that experiential learning is far more concerned with **self concept** than are other sorts of learning. Any activity that involves "personal learning" must, by definition, involve a sense of self. When we modify or change something personal, we modify or change our sense of who we are (Knowles 1978). Many students found role play particularly difficult and embarrassing to take part in. The complaint was also made that such role plays could be "unreal". Role play, by its format, requires people to "pretend" and to "act", rather as though they were in a play. The point about actors in a play is that they are not being themselves but acting as though they were other people. Given the students' emphasis on clinical learning, on learning from real life and on personal learning, it may be the case that role play in nurse education must give way to activities that offer a greater opportunity to reflect on **real life** clinical situations. In this study was the students often felt that they learned a considerable amount about nursing from observing **role models**. In other words, the real-life role was more acceptable than was role play. This emphasis on role modelling in the clinical setting has been exploited as a teaching method by Walsh, VandenBosch and Boehm (1989) who argue that an important way to teach excellent nursing practice is to ensure that it is model in clinical placements. They also suggest that exemplary role modelling is one means of bridging the theory-practice gap in nursing.

Recently, a number of writers have described the use of the experiential learning cycle in helping learners to extract meaning from their clinical work through reflection and discussion groups in those clinical areas (Iwasiw and Sleightholm-Cairns 1990, Quinsland and Van Ginkel 1984, Reilly and Oermann 1985). Clarke has also advocated nursing developing reflective skills as the means of making considered clinical judgements (Clarke 1986). Clarke and Feltham (1990) have suggested that students may help each other to reflect on their nursing practice by the process known as "peer teaching", as has Costello (1989). Also, there is a growing literature on the role of the mentor, supervisor or preceptor in clinical settings as a person who not only counsels and supports students but who also helps them to process their learning (Rolfe 1990, Donovan 1990, Bracken and Davis 1989, Barber and Norman 1987).

Most of the respondents indicated that experiential learning could be fun to take part in. There are a number of possibilities here. First, it is possible that people enjoy taking part in activities that involve participation. Rogers (1967, 1983), Freire (1972) Kolb (1984) and Jarvis (1987) have discussed the need for people to take part, actively, in the learning process. Second, learning situations that involve activity have a less predictable outcome than do learning activities such as the lecture. In the lecture, the teacher controls the learning situation to a considerable degree in terms of outcomes, process, and student involvement. When students are actively involved in the learning situation, there can be less prediction of outcome and structure because the people participating in the activity will all experience that activity in various and different ways. This can lead to a sense of "the unknown", which could heighten curiosity and enjoyment levels.

It is possible that the Von Restorff effect (Palmer and Pope 1984) could operate in these sorts of circumstances. The Von Restorff effect refers to the fact that we tend to learn things when they are presented in dramatic and "different" ways. If, for example, a student had been used to learning session being mostly of the lecture variety, the introduction of experiential learning activities could heighten learning because those activities were "different". Presumably, too, the fact that those activities were different could lead to a greater level of enjoyment through variation of routine. A longer term study would have to be implemented to identify whether or not experiential learning methods are **more effective** methods of learning and whether or not the enjoyment factor was sustained with constant use of the method.

What is it useful for?

Educational activities do not have to have a utility value. Peters (1972) for example, argues that an educational experience may be of value for its own sake and that to seek the practical use of every educational activity is to take a narrow view of what it means to be educated. On the other hand, what is under discussion, here, is education and **training** to a practical end : the development of nursing practitioners who can register as nurses at the end of the course. Therefore it is reasonable to ask what the value is of activities taken part in during a nursing course. Two outcomes of the experiential learning process were identified by most respondents in this study. They were :
- Experiential learning can increase self-awareness,
- Experiential learning can aid the development of interpersonal skills.

Here, again, we see the issue of personal learning emerging. As was noted above, any activities that make you question your own stock of personal knowledge are likely to affect your sense of self. Many respondents felt that experiential learning could enhance self-awareness. This is certainly in accord with current suggestions about the value of experiential learning in this domain (Kagan, Kay and

Evans 1986, Kenworthy and Nicklin 1989, Burnard 1990). All of these writers have stressed that in order to develop self-awareness, learners must take an active part in the learning process. You cannot, it would seem, learn about yourself in a detached way : you must be involved.

The idea of self-awareness links directly with that of reflection, discussed above. To become self-aware involves in at least a minimal amount of inward reflection. To come to know "who you are" first involves reflecting on what is going on "inside". On the other hand, the concept of "self-awareness" is a slippery one. The tutors in the interviews in this study had difficulty in defining what they meant by self-awareness and the literature on the topic is large and diverse. It ranges from theories of self in psychological terms (Kelly 1955, Bannister and Fransella 1986), to theories of self in philosophical terms (Sartre 1956) to spiritual and "transpersonal" theories (Wilber 1981, Rowan 1989) to biological theories (Ginsburg 1984) There is no consensus of agreement as to what we are to understand by the concept of "self" and therefore the concept of "self-awareness" is likely to remain rather vague. The recent literature in nursing on the topic, has generally argued, however, that self-awareness is a "good thing" for nurses (Bond 1986, Burnard 1990). It has usually suggested that such awareness is necessary for nurses if they are to begin to understand and help other people. Whether or not this is actually the case remains the subject of further research.

Experiential learning methods have also been widely recommended as the vehicle for learning about interpersonal skills in nursing (Reynolds 1985, Reynolds and Cormack 1987, Marshfield 1985, Raichura 1987, Burnard 1990). Again, the characteristics of personal involvement, personal learning and reflecting on experience are all widely mooted as those that facilitate the development of such skills. The findings of this study support the notion that experiential learning methods are useful for learning interpersonal skills. It is encouraging, too, that interpersonal skills were so widely discussed in the study, given that the formal study of such skills is a fairly recent addition to most nursing syllabi.

What "type" of experiential learning are nurses involved in?

Weil and McGill (1989) suggested that there were four "types" of experiential learning practitioners and these have been discussed in chapter one. Briefly, the four types were as follows :

Type one: The assessment and accreditation of prior learning through the process of living : job experience, life experience and so forth.

Type two: Experiential learning focused on change in higher and continuing eduction.

Type three: Experiential learning as a process of social change.

Type four: Personal growth and development : the "humanistic" approach.

Reviewing these four types of experiential learning and the data from respondents in this study, it became clear that the type that many of the educators (and particularly those in psychiatric nurse education) could be grouped under was type four : experiential learning concerned with personal growth and development - the humanistic approach. This was made particularly evident when the tutors being interviewed were asked to identify writers that they felt had influenced their experiential learning practice : Carl Rogers and John Heron (both humanistic writers) were often mentioned. This affiliation with one particular school of thought has its problems as we shall explore in the second level analysis offered below.

The Tutors Perceptions

The tutors in the interview section of this study tended to discuss experiential learning in terms of activities that they were involved in the school or college of nursing. This suggests that the focus of the tutors" world of work is the school rather than the clinical setting.

The Students' Perceptions

The students in this study mostly related experiential learning to the idea of learning in the clinical setting. This is a similar finding to that of Harvey and Vaughan (1990). In a study of 203 student nurses in which they used the Osgood semantic differential scale to explore students' attitudes towards various learning and teaching methods, Harvey and Vaughan found that nurses learn from practical clinical activities, by observing role models and by interacting with people.

They found, too, that students did not have a favourable attitude towards lecturers.

In the present study, the emphasis, from the students' point of view was on learning in the clinical setting rather than learning in the classroom. On the other hand, the study contrasts with Dux' study of 13 nurse educators in which she found that the lecture method was still the favoured teaching and learning method in general nurse education (Dux 1989). In a study of 107 general nursing students, O'Kell (1988) found that both general and psychiatric nursing students preferred the lecture method to experiential learning methods, although the general students ranked experiential learning methods far lower in terms of popularity than did the psychiatric nursing students. Dux' and O'Kell's studies focused on the **school** teaching and learning methods. What is notable in the present study is that students were suggesting that they learnt best in the clinical setting. Indeed, a number of the students in the interview section of the study were scathing about their experience of the school of nursing and most were adamant that they learned more in the clinical setting than they did in the school. Perhaps educators would do well to focus their attention more on improving the learning environment in the clinical setting than on enhancing teaching and learning methods in the colleges and schools.

Second Level Analysis

So far, the level of analysis has focused on the explicit : what was expressed by the interviewees and the questionnaire respondents. The aim, throughout, was to focus on what the respondents had said. Now, the level of analysis moves to a more abstract level. For this form of analysis, it was important to "stand back" from the interview transcripts and the literature in an attempt to identify some of the "processes" occurring within those two media. Two categories emerged out of this standing back process. The first can be described as "learning the language", the second as "learning the values". Those two categories are now described.

Learning the Language

What became apparent when reviewing the literature, particularly on the humanistic approach to experiential learning and related topics, that the humanistic school of thinkers and writers tend to adopt a particular "language style". That language style can be divided into two aspects, the first of which I shall call "Alternative Style", the second of which I will call "Existentialese". These two aspects of a language style ran through much of the writing on the topic and was sometimes found in the transcripts of the tutors and students interviews. These two aspects of language style will now be discussed.

Language Style I : "Alternative Style"

This is a style of language used most frequently in certain writings in the sixties but which also grew out of a previous generation of slang that may be associated with a bohemian or "outsider" (Wilson 1956) lifestyle. A very extreme version of it would be the following quotation from Lipton (1960) :

> "She's square" the young man told me afterward.
> "She **knows** all about it -up here-" tapping his forehead -
> but she doesn't dig it man. Like you got to swing **with**
> it or you get hung up... (Lipton 1960 : 24)

This is particular characteristic of the style : a novel use of words ("dig", "hung up") that come to be regular currency amongst a particular group of a society, usually the younger members.From that extreme, it is possible to identify other examples of the use of slang in the humanistic literature. This, for example, in a book called Humanistic Teaching :

> Socrates said : "Know thyself" and today's dedicated,
> young "groovy" teacher says : "Do your own thing".
> (Clark and Kadis 1971 : 4).

A particularly pertinent example would be the "Gestalt Prayer" written by Frit Perls, founder of Gestalt Therapy (Perls 1973). A number of the tutors interviewed either mentioned Perls as an

226

influence or discussed their use of Gestalt approaches to experiential learning. Masson (1990) has this to say about the prayer :

> It is hard to hear the famous Gestalt Prayer with which Perls began his group sessions...without a twinge of embarrassment. It would be trite at any time, but seems particularly wedded to the 1960's. (Masson 1990 : 60).

Perls' prayer reads as follows and exactly sums up the notion of Alternative Style :

> I do my thing, and you do your thing.
> I am not in this world to live up to your expectations.
> And you are not in this world to live up to mine.
> You are you and I am I,
> And if by chance we find each other,
> it's beautiful,
> If not, it can't be helped.
> (Perls 1973 : 3).

The **values** that are expressed are not under discussion, at present, merely the use of language.

Such language was perhaps in common usage during the "hippy" period of the 1960's and is certainly most noticeable in writings of that time (Hudson 1983). However, it is still evident in more recent work in the humanistic field. Sometimes, the allusion to the 60's is made explicit, as in the following extract from a paper on psychodrama in Self and Society : The European Journal of Humanistic Psychology, which combines both the use of Language Style I ("The Open Centre is a space where...") and the acknowledgement of the writer's roots :

> The Open Centre is a space where I feel at home, free of the rule of fear governing many people's working lives. Here I am at 44, after much effort to avoid a career, a shameless, ageing hippy...(Gladstone 1990 : 24).

The language is also reflected in many of the publications that are heavily referred to in the nursing literature on experiential learning approaches (see, for example, Kilty 1983, Bond and Kilty

1983, Heron 1982, Rowan 1988). This, in turn, seems to have filtered through to workers in the field and is to be found in some of the interview transcripts. Examples of the use of this language style in those interviews are as follows :

> "I see experiential learning as very here-and-now and
> focusing on that in the learning encounter."

Here we find the reference to the "here-and-now" which can be found throughout the literature on humanistic psychology and was very much the central focus of many of the 60's psychotherapies (Rowan 1988). Also, the use of the term "learning encounter" perhaps reflects back to the "encounter culture" (Schutz 1967, 1971, Rogers 1970) of that period. The interviewee who is quoted here went on to discuss the influence of "encounter groups".

> "I'm actually doing the heavy stuff now."

It is suggested that this represents a similar use of slang. From the context from which it is taken, the "heavy stuff" appears to mean that the interviewee was currently engaged on a course which allowed him to explore the "deeper" aspects of himself, through the use of catharsis and emotional release (the word "heavy" is used in this way by Rowan 1988 to describe such methods). Again, both the word "heavy" and the accent on catharsis is very much a reflection of the 60's culture of free expression and self-development. The same respondent went on to use the phrase :

> "...which is easy when I want to do my own thing but at
> the same time I want to accommodate you..."

The idea of "doing your own thing" reflects straight back to Perl"s "prayer" and to the 60's notion of independence and free thinking. Along similar lines, another respondent suggested that a particular experiential learning activity meant that :

> "The power is with the client."

"Power to the People" was a popular slogan in the 1960's and reflected the anticipated "quiet revolution" that was thought, by some to be occurring at the time and the development of a "counter culture

(Roszak 1969). Heron"s writing on experiential learning sometimes reflected this anticipated revolution. Writing of the use of a particular style of counselling, Heron suggested that :

> To try to help prematurely the worst victims of the old system will forever subvert the establishment of a viable alternative system. (Heron 1978 : 24)

Exactly what the "old system" and the "alternative systems" were, is not made clear by Heron. As we have noted throughout this book, Heron's work has influenced a number of writers on experiential learning in nursing.

Many of the tutors used the term "workshop" to describe the type of structure they gave to learning situations and the word is widely used in the literature on experiential learning (Knowles 1978, Heron 1972, Burnard 1985, Heron 1979a etc). One commentator links its usage firmly with the 1960's "alternative society", offering the following definition and an example of its use :

> **Workshop.** Any form of group activity involving study or discussion. The term is much used by members of the Alternative Society and the Left generally, mainly no doubt because it sounds busy and productive and gives mere talk the cachet of solid manual work - [e.g] *"The fluid situation of largely unprepared workshops did not alienate many people" (Spare Rib, April, 1975)* (Hudson 1983 : 194).

Other examples of the language style under discussion and drawn from the interviews with the tutors are as follows :

"I always make sure I **check it out** with the audience".

"We haven't really **got it together** yet."

"It's the **person-orientation : I love it**"

"I think it [experiential learning] **really rhymed** with my personality"

"What I do then is **just let it happen.**"

This question of a style of language has implications for the ways in which tutors and, to a lesser extent, students may view the world in which they work, teach and learn. Postman and Weingartner (1969) reporting on the work of Sapir and Whorf report as follows :

> [Whorf and Sapir's] studies of the language systems of different cultures led them to the conclusion...that each language - including both its structure and its lexicon represented a unique way of perceiving reality. They believed that we are imprisoned, so to speak, in a house of language. We try to assess what is outside the house from our position within it. However, the house is oddly shaped (and no one knows precisely what a normal shape would be). There is a limited number of windows. The windows are tinted and are at odd angles. We have no choice but to see what the structure of the house permits us to see. (Postman and Weingartner 1969 : 42).

Boudieu (1971) supports this application of Sapir and Whorf's work to the field of **styles** of language as well as to the language itself when he writes :

> What is usually known as the Sapir-Whorf hypobook is perhaps never so satisfactorily applicable as to intellectual life; words, **and especially figures of speech** and figures of thought that are characteristic of a school of thought, mould thought as much as they express it. Linguistic and intellectual patterns are all the more important in determining what individuals take as worthy of being though and what they think of it in that they operate outside all critical awareness. [emphasis added] (Boudieu 1971 : 195).

The structure of the language used by the humanistic experiential learning writers might, therefore, like all other styles of language, be **limiting** their perceptions. If, to continue the argument, students learn or partly learn that language style as part of the learning process, then those students may be blinkered by the words. A second point, is that the language used is a **dated** one and this may have implications for the credibility of tutors if they use the style of language with a group of students for whom it is dated.

Also, on this issue of style, Huges (1988) in his analysis of the development of social development of language, describes a :

> ...word field reflecting the moralization of value-terms which are imprecise or directionless, such as **progress, relevance, concern, commitment,** and **awareness.** (Huges 1988 : 86)

He goes on to suggest that :

> Style, rather than content, is the aspect stress in **cool, laid back,** and **uptight.** (Huges 1988 : 86)

Perhaps the exponents of the Alternative style are offering just that a style - rather than a tightly argued set of theories and concepts. That style may firmly root them in a particular part of a particular age : the 1960's.

Not that the use of a particular style of language in this field is as recent, even, as the 1960's. More than forty years ago, Barron and Krulee (1948) reported the acknowledgement of words in this way in the field of interpersonal skills training. Barron and Krullee were describing the running of an interpersonal skills laboratory (one of the National Skills Laboratories, associated with the father of the "T" or training group, Kurt Lewin [Aronson1980]) in Bethel on the East Coast of the US. They noted that :

> Reaction to the many new or unusual words which were being used in the laboratory, "Bethelesque" as they came to be called, began to be expressed in a way that persisted throughout the laboratory program : "change-agent", "involvement", "out group" and the like..."
> (Barron and Krulee 1948 : 15).

Noticeable in Barron and Krullee's account of their interpersonal workshop in the 40's is the similarity in the use of language used for identifying the goals of their workshop. Their goals could easily have been drawn from a late 1980's nurses' interpersonal skills workshop :

1. Increased understanding on a verbal level of underlying principles of dealing with people.

2. Increased sensitivity to and awareness of those dynamic interactions between people in groups that are relevant to the diagnosis of human relation situations.
3. Skills in actually using this understanding.
4. Increased awareness of one's own motivation and increased self-awareness. The faculty felt that self-understanding was essential in working with others. (Barron and Krullee 1948 : 12).

This extract contains many of the aspects of language that carried over through the 50's, 60's and 70's and found their way into 1980's nurses training courses : "human relation situations", "increase awareness of one"s own motivation and increased self-awareness." Arguably, though, the style of language became "sharpened" in the 60's when the particular sorts of slang such as "where you're at" and "doing your own thing" became incorporated into everyday speech in a way that it had not previously been (Hudson 1983). Indeed, it is possible to map the development of this language style through four decades. Figure 12.3 the path of such development.

The diagram illustrates the development of humanistic psychology and examples of the language style. Arguably, from the 1970's, nursing theory and nursing education began to absorb some of these principles both in the form of nursing theory and curriculum development (ENB 1982). It seems possible that the language style associated with humanistic psychology was also adopted to some degree and thus became part of the language of nursing education - particularly the experiential learning approach to nurse education, which leant so heavily on humanistic psychology.

Decade	Developments	Example of Language Style from the Period.
1940's - 1950's	Beginning of the 'T' group movement and of Humanistic Psychology	"Change agent", "involvement", "out group". (Barron and Krulee 1948).
1950's - 1960's	Development of Humanistic psychology and of a range of "alternative" therapies (gestalt, encounter etc.)	"Like you got to swing with it or get hung up." (Lipton 1960)
1960's - 1970's	Incorporation of some humanistic themes into mainstream education.	"I do my thing, you do your thing" (Perls 1973)
1970's - 1980's	Development of humanistic principles into nursing and nurse education. The development of experiential learning.	"Actions taken [by a group leader] should not cause a student to feel "put down"... (Tomlinson 1985).

Figure 12.3 Development of Stages of Development of Humanistic Psychology and the Parallel development of the Language Style

233

Another explanation for the continuance of this particular language style in nursing education is that tutors take some years to get to the point where they train as tutors. To undertake tutor training is to have completed at least three years as a registered nurse. Undertaking tutor training also usually requires secondment by a health authority. Typically, people coming to such courses are in their late twenties or early thirties. Such people may have "brought with them" the language style from the 60's or may be receptive to it when they read it or hear it in teacher training colleges. To continue this regress, those teachers in training colleges may well be influenced in the same ways. Finally, those writing books about the topic of humanistic psychology and humanistic approaches to experiential learning may also be products of the 1960's.

An important part of using language in this way, is that the user must be **credible** in using it. The idea of being in role in order to use a particular style of language was reinforced during a recent conversation with my adolescent son, after I had tried to use some of the slang that he used with his friends. His suggestion was :

"You shouldn't even try, because even when you get the right words, it still doesn't sound right".

"Why?"

"Because you're too old and you're my father."

Or, as Bernstein put it : "If you cannot manage the role, you can't produce the appropriate speech" (Bernstein 1972 p166). The tutors that have learned to use this language may sometimes lack credibility. When they **have** also found credibility, they may win converts in the form of students, who also begin to adopt the language. In turn, a sense of community and like-mindedness develops. The language style marks you out as "one who knows". The language style serves to tell others that you are "one of them". As Trudgill 1983) points out, language styles not only serve to communicate **content** but also serve as "identification markers" : they allow others to quickly come to know more about you. Trudgill suggests that :

> ...whenever we speak we cannot avoid giving our listeners clues about our origins and the sort of person we are. (Trudgill 1983 : 14).

It may be argued that this need to be marked out in a particular way is more pressing in the psychiatric nursing domain than it is in the general. The psychiatric community is a minority one in the nursing profession. Until recently, its focus has been the large institution which has been characterised by a closed, inward-looking approach (Goffman 1961). The nursing hierarchy is also rather more relaxed in the psychiatric hospital than it is in the general. It is possible that the use of a particular language style could serve as a means of identification between colleagues and "carers" in the institutional setting. Given that psychiatric nurses often do not wear uniforms and may need to separate off the "them" of the patients with the "us" of the staff, this language style may help the staff to maintain their seperateness.

It may also serve to bind together **therapists** in such a setting, for the language style that has been described here, is also to be found in the psychotherapy and counselling literature (Kopp 1972, Egan 1977, Tschudin 1986). The language style may give the therapists a common mode of communication between themselves - a "shorthand" for conveying therapeutic ideas. It may also gloss over some of the problems that psychotherapy and counselling have still to address squarely : the most important one being whether or not psychotherapy and counselling actually **help**. The language may help to convey a sense of authority and wisdom in a field where there are still many unknowns and, possibly, imponderables.

Finally, in this area, the language may help to pass on the **values** associated with the counselling and psychotherapy field - notably those of the client-centred approach. As we have noted, the language style occurs frequently in the humanistic literature but probably less often in the fields of behavioural and psychodynamic therapies. In this way, the person who uses the language not only conveys, quickly, that she is of a humanistic and client-centred orientation, but also indicates that it is likely that she endorses many of the values that go with that movement : the importance of freedom of choice, the value of client choice and so forth. The language style becomes the culture carrier (Fox 1975).

An analysis of the transcripts of the **students'** interviews did not reveal the use of a similar langauge style. Instead, their language style was more **personal** and had a there was a tendency to use "fillers" such as "like I said"; "you could say" and "well..." Examples of this personalised style are as follows :

" Well, its like I said, it's just dealing with the people more than the facts."

"Well, you could say that role playing in a classroom is experiential learning - you could say that."

"Well, like I said, it does sort of reproduce a sort of situation..."

"Not really, not in my experience. I mean, when we've like done role plays..."

This style of speaking is reminiscent of Bernstein's "restricted code" (Bernstein 1972) with its dependence on the use of the personal accounts and on the pronoun "I". Bernstein also noted the frequent use of tags such as "wouldn"t it?" and "aren't they", which were present in the students' transcripts. Ironically, the students all talked more of **their own experience** and used the word "I" more frequently than did the tutors. The irony is that one of the tutors most frequent notions was that experiential learning was about **personal experience** and yet it was the students who personalised their interviews.

Bernstein also described "elaborated code" or the use of a style of language that was more formal and did not rely on the use of personal pronouns but more on detailed argument. Whilst the tutors often offered detailed arguments of their points of view, they also used "I" fairly frequently but did not use the "tags" of "like I said", or "it does sort of", in the way that the students did. It is suggested, therefore, that whilst the students appeared to use "restricted code" fairly frequently, the tutors did not use "elaborated code very often but neither did they use "restricted code". The point, here, is that both groups appeared to be **talking in different styles**. In summary : the tutors often used language styles I and II (described below), whilst the students often used "restricted code". The question is : do these two styles of communication make a difference to shared meanings between the two groups and/or do they inhibit communication between the two?

236

Language Style II : Existentialese

Linked to the above style, is the other aspect of the style which I have called "existentialese". This refers to the use of language in a particular way and which is concerned with existential notions such as "self", "being", "becoming" and so forth. The literature on humanistic approaches to care, teaching and experiential learning contains passages which use these concepts in such a way as to **convey the impression that they mean something** but whose meaning is not always clear. Two examples of this style of writing can be offered to illustrate the concept of "existentialese". Both are from writers in nursing.

> To say "you" to a person is to acknowledge that person, affirm the other, believe the other, trust the other without reserve, simply because the other **is**. (Tschudin 1986 : 7).

> Personal knowledge is concerned with the knowing, encountering and actualising of the concrete, individual self. (Carper 1978 : 28)

Although it is not clear, it appears that Tschudin has written as though the English language had a personal as well as an impersonal form of "you", as in the French "tu" and "vous". As English does not, the statement is meaningless. To take this point further : if English **did** have a personal form of "you", the above statement would still be begging many questions. It cannot be assumed that because you use a "familiar" style of address or greeting, that you are **necessarily** implying all of the things that Tschudin suggests that you might be.

Carper's statement is equally difficult to penetrate. The concept of 'self' is an abstraction : to talk about a "concrete self" is to use words in a curious way. Also, what it means to engage in "knowing, encountering and actualising" such a self is not clear.

Both writers presumably **meant** something by both of these statements but what they mean is not made clear.

The two extracts are typical of the style that I have called "existentialese" is that it not only uses existential concepts but the "tone" of the writing seems to be suggesting something affirmative and positive. What that "something" is, is never made explicit.

Another example comes from the humanistic psychology literature and is perhaps even more obscure :

> The immediate content of our experience is void of meaning for it can never point away from itself. It doesn't "mean" anything since, by virtue of its very being or suchness, it is meaning. It is always unique, a cosmic "one-off" as it were, focused on the individual consciousness. (Pankhurst 1987 :138)

Sometimes the style can take on a rather quaint form as in the following example from Kilty's Experiential Learning (1983). Kilty was discussing the need for training in the field of experiential learning and cautions that :

> Some of the methods do invite learners to reconsider some of their more deeply held characteristic ways of being. (Kilty 1983 :13)

There were various examples of the use of existentialese offered by tutors during their interviews. For the sake of brevity, two examples are offered here. Both illustrate the use of a positive style linked to the use of existential words.

> **Example One** : You have to experience life to meet life. Whether you are actively participating or not, you are experiencing life, so to live is to experience it.

> **Example Two** : Because when you start to loosen experientially, the cognitive part of things, you look at it properly. You have had the background, you have grown with the feeling.

In both examples, too, there are hints of the Language Style II, described above : "to live is to experience it" and "you have grown with the feeling". Again, what is to be understood by the statements is not made explicit.

The criticism may be levelled that all of these examples are "bleeding chunks", divorced from their context. The examples have been chosen, however, because even when they are read in context, the reader is offered no "way in" to the meanings intended by the writer or the speaker. There seems to be a certain hypnotic element involved too : there is an illusion that something is being read or heard. During the interviews from which the two extracts are drawn, the interviewer recalls no problems with understanding what was being said at the time. It was only when the interviews were transcribed and the words transferred to paper, that the puzzle occurred.

The immediate problems with existentialese is that it represents a breakdown in communication. Many, complex issues such as "self", "experience" and "knowledge" can be glossed over through the use of colourful but "empty" language. Issues that are inherently problematic are not treated as problematic but as resolved in some way. Again, if students are being presented with such existentialese, there is the possibility of their being "hypnotised" in the same way. This "hypnotism" may also be explained through Boudieu's (1971) reference, above, that "linguistic patterns,,,operate outside all critical awareness". Thus the person who is hearing those sorts of words and who is immersed in the style of talking and writing, no longer seeks to filter out the sound from the unsound, the logical from the illogical : the style of communication becomes the expected. Critical faculties are suspended because the "critical antennae" are no longer operating. This could also have been operating during the interviews : the interviewer was unable to both listen and analyse what was being said and was "unaware" of the linguistic patterns that were being used because he was both immersed in it and critically unaware of what was being said.

Acquiring the Values

Another issue, linked to the issue of learning the language, is that a variety of particular values are involved in many of the writings on experiential learning. Rogers (1983) for example, makes it clear that he believes that people are essentially "good" and left to their own devices can make the "right" choices for themselves. This point of view is summed up by Rogers as follows :

> ...the innermost core of man's nature, the deepest layers of his personality, the base of his 'animal nature' is positive in nature - is basically socialised, forward-moving, rational and realistic. (Rogers 1967 : 36).

This theme of inherent goodness can be viewed as a reaction to the Freudian view of persons as essentially bad and to the Christian ethic of people as essentially evil (Murphy and Kovach 1972). In Rogers' case, it is made clear in his biography (Kirschenbaum 1982) that Rogers, in deciding that people were essential "good", was reacting to an early training for preparation to enter the Church. According to his biographer, Rogers as a young man came to question his religious beliefs and then to reject them, preferring to view persons' as both essentially good and as responsible, to some degree, for their own actions.

Other values that are frequently identified in the literature on the humanistic approach to experiential learning are : that students should be self-directing (Rogers 1952, 1983, Maslow 1972), that people can and should be involved in "personal growth" (Heron 1977a, Rowan 1988) and that expression of emotion is a "good thing" (Heron 1977a, Rowan 1988,). Perhaps the most explicit attempt at formalising such values is the one made by Jones (1990) in his proposal for a Humanistic Creed. He suggests that the creed had been "derived from the literature on humanistic psychology and from the way that humanistic psychologists tend to work". The points of the creed are as follows :

I believe in :

* the validation of choice in lifestyles, whether or not it is approved by established power groups in society,

* recognition of wants, needs and desires,

* a disciplined method for personal growth,

* autonomy and cooperation in relationships,

* authoritative guides as opposed to authoritarian ones,

* the empowerment of clients and not the control of patients and cases,

* validation of emotion and emotional competence,

* experiential learning. (Jones 1990 : 4)

What is interesting about this list is its use of quasi- religious tones in its formulation as a "Creed". This is particularly interesting given humanistic psychology's usual insistence on the centrality of the "person" and of "free choice". Also, it is rather odd that Jones is suggesting experiential learning as an article of faith. This evangelising element of humanistic psychology is also present in its dismissal of other psychologies as somehow not acceptable or just plain wrong. In a discussion about psychodynamic, behavioural, and cognitive psychology, Rowan (1988) dismisses them all as follows :

> So it is clear how humanistic psychology would reject psychoanalysis and behaviourism. But how would it reject the third form of psychology which has come up in the past ten years and which now dominates academia - cognitive psychology? Cognitive psychology is perhaps ԱՈՈՀ Ու the greatest con tricks ever perpetrated (Rowan 1988 : 54)

As we have seen earlier in this report, this sort of dramatic statement is not new in humanistic writing. It will be recalled that Moreno, for example, talked of "teaching people to play God" (Moreno 1977). What seems to permeate some of the writing in the humanistic field is its certainty that it has "got things right", combined with a disregard for traditional research methods. Reason and Rowan (1981) regard traditional methods as "old paradigm". The humanistic movement does seem to have an evangelical zeal about it and has been described by one commentator (Wallis 1984) as an example of an "elementary form of the new religious life", thus developing Durkheim's original work.

The humanistic psychology approach to experiential learning has been very evident in both the nursing literature and in the data collected in this study - particularly in the data collected from nurse tutors. This humanistic bias may lead to a clash in values between those developed during the 1960's and those of the early 1990's. Writing of the development of humanistic psychology in counselling, Woolfe, Dryden and Charles-Edwards (1989) have this to say :

> The object of person-centred counselling...is to help the client "to become what he/she is capable of becoming" {Rogers 1951}, or, to employ an even more well-worn phrase associated with Maslow, to achieve self-

actualisation {Maslow 1962}. These terms have a slightly hollow ring about them in the enterprise economy of the late 1980s in Britain, in which the division between the "haves" and the "have nots" is sharply apparent. Striving for self-actualisation is easier if one is well-off, well-housed, has a rewarding and secure job and lives in a pleasant environment than if one is unemployed, poor, ill-housed, and lives in a run-down neighbourhood. Terms like self-actualisation simply do not feature in and do not derive from the culture of the 1980s. (Woolfe, Dryden and Charles-Edwards 1989 : 10)

Howard made a similar point rather more directly when, discussing the changing needs of clients who seek counselling, suggested about counsellors that :

It is time we shed our naivety and the "syrupy" illusions of Carl Rogers and his many cohorts. (Howard 1990 : 15)

These writers raise important questions that relate to issues in this study. There have been considerable changes in life in the UK since the 1960's. The political climate has changed, employment patterns and patterns of health and sickness have also changed, some would say irreversibly (Bowen 1990). Ashton and Seymour (1988) sum up some of these changes as follows :

Fundamental changes are taking place both in the way we view ill-health and the way as individuals, families and governments response to it. In the United Kingdom ministerial reputations and careers are being made and lost out of the health-related issues of AIDS, drugs, heart disease and the environmental conditions of the inner cities. The once sacred National Health Service is under attack for failing to deliver the goods and the long assumed immunity to accountability of physicians is falling away week by week. In Liverpool, 26 per cent of adult men are unemployed and nationally the infant mortality rate has just risen for the first time in 16 years. (Ashton and Seymour 1989 : vii).

Murgatroyd and Woolfe (1982) note that approaches to counselling and caring for people with different problems of living are also changing. They suggest that there has been a move away from the client-centred approach of Rogers towards an interest in short-term, crisis-oriented counselling for which more directive, action-oriented procedures are usually advocated. The question that can be addressed towards the findings from this study is this : are the values being espoused by nurse educators in the early 1990's and expressed through their educational language, reflecting values that are up to thirty years behind the times? Nurse education, like any vocational preparation, is a social enterprise that cannot be divorced from the social, economic and political environment in which it is practised. There is some evidence, in this study, to suggest that such a divorce may exist and that nurse educators need to review that values that lie behind their practices if they are not to be seen as purveyors of outdated values.

The Users and Recipients of Experiential Learning : Two Profiles

In drawing together the themes that have emerged out of this study, it is possible to identify two broad types of users and receivers of experiential learning. These are illustrated in the two profiles in figure 11.3. It is not suggested that these are "ideal types" but they do represent features that were frequently present in the two groups' interviews and they do suggest different ways of thinking about experiential learning.

Cultural Isogloss

It is possible to develop a theory of a "cultural isogloss" exiting between nurse tutors and students in the field of experiential learning. An isogloss is the line of demarcation between two languages (Greek: "iso" = "same; "gloss" = "tongue"). Thus, a line may be drawn between Holland and Germany, where one language finishes and another begins. Such a line is not clear and distinct but it does exist. So to, it may be suggested that a language and values barrier exists between the tutors and students. The tutors speak a different style of language and embrace a different set of values to the students. The two groups have different views of the "point" of experiential learning and of the educational process itself. This cultural isogloss may be the thing that gets in the way of learning in the school setting. More than just a "generation gap" it may help to explain how students become alienated from the school, albeit unconsciously. The two groups of people are separated from each other by different language styles but possibly, also, by different **understandings** of the words involved. Further, the two groups do not seem to necessarily understand or appreciate the perceptions of each other. Figure 12.4 summarises some of the issues from this chapter regarding the differences between students and tutors perceptions.

	The Educator	C U L T U R A L I S O L L O S S	The Student
Life world	The school or college of nursing		The clinical setting
Focus of the learning process	The individual and his or her personal experience		Learning how to be a nurse.
Aim of the learning process	Self-awareness and the development of interpersonal skills		Learning about nursing.
Style of Language	Styles I and II		Restricted code
Experiential learning methods experienced.	Role play, structured group activities, pairs exercises, etc.		

Figure 12.4 Differences of Perception : Tutors and Students

Recommendations

Recommendations from a descriptive study must necessarily be tentative. The findings of such a study may not be generalised out to a larger sample. Another study with other respondents could yield different findings. This is likely to be true, too, of studies that use random or larger samples, given the complexity of human beings and the variability of their experience. The recommendations that derive from this study may be categorised as follows :

- Those concerning the use and structuring of experiential learning,
- Those concerning the nature of the tutor and student experience in nurse education,
- Those concerning the language and values associated with experiential learning,
- Those concerning further research.

Structuring Experiential Learning

A number of the respondents found experiential learning methods to be embarrassing to take part in. Also, the tutors often worried about whether or not experiential learning sessions could get out of control and whether or not the activities might provoke an emotional response in their students that they (the tutors) could not handle. Further, the students often noted that role play could be difficult to take part in. Finally, many of the students acknowledge the primacy of clinical work in learning about nursing. The recommendations that can be made here, then, are these :

- Experiential learning methods used in the training of nurses should be ones that respect the dignity of the students,
- Such methods should be ones that allow the students to withdraw if they feel emotionally threatened by them,
- The methods should be grounded in the students' **clinical experience**. Experiential learning activities should always reflect clinical practice and not become "islands of experience".
- Tutors should receive sufficient training in the use of experiential learning methods to enable them to cope with contingencies such as emotional release, with confidence.

Tutor and Student Experience in Nurse Education

As with a number of other studies (Alexander 1983, Ogier 1982), this study highlighted a gap between the "school" and the "clinical" setting. Frequently, the students felt that the place where they "really" learned about nursing was in the clinical situation, working alongside other nurses. The recommendation, here, then, is that tutors pursue methods of enabling the school/clinical gap to be narrowed. Ironically, it could be possible for the use of experiential learning approaches to **widen** that gap. It appears that some tutors, particularly in the psychiatric nursing field, develop an interest and expertise in the use of school-based experiential learning methods such as role play or psychodrama. Success with these methods may mean that such tutors decrease the amount of time they spend in clinical settings whilst they develop and use that expertise. The knack must be to find ways of incorporating the skills of experiential learning facilitation with clinical learning. Primary nursing and the development of the lecturer practitioner (Bond 1990, Wright 1990) are two recent attempts at bridging the theory/practice gap. Others should be explored.

Language and Values

It has been suggested in this discussion that distinctive language styles are used in the humanistic literature relating to experiential learning and there were indications that such language was used by some of the tutors in the study. It was noted, too, that certain values could be associated with the use of experiential learning. It is suggested that such language and value systems could clash with those of the students who undertake experiential learning activities and that writers and practitioners in the field of nurse education may wish to pay attention to the language that they use both to describe the philosophy of the experiential learning approach and in their practice as facilitators or teachers of nursing.

Further Research

This study has attempted to clarify what experiential learning means to tutors and students in nursing. The next step must be to find out

247

the degree to which such learning and teaching methods contribute to nursing care. If the aim of nurse education is to produce confident and skilled nursing practitioners, then the methods used to train and educate them must be effective. The next stage, then, is to test the efficacy of some of these methods. Research is never a closed cycle of activities. As usual in research, this study has raised a variety of questions about the process of learning to be a nurse and about the role of the educator in that process.

Constraints of time mean that a research project has to stop somewhere. It would have been interesting to explore the language issue further and the researcher has plans to explore the use of language in the humanistic literature via a detailed content analysis.

Final Summary

This study has illustrated the perceptions of some tutors and students regarding experiential learning. It has noted that both groups tended to see experiential learning as being concerned with learning by doing and through reflection. They also felt that it was both fun to take part in and yet embarrassing. Both groups felt that experiential learning activities were useful for learning interpersonal skills and for developing self awareness. The theoretical and practical implications of these findings have been discussed.

A tentative theory of two "language styles" has also been developed and the suggestion has been made that such language styles may, at times, stand between tutors and students. As ever, more work needs to be done on all fronts. The project, like most others, raises as many questions as it answers.

Appendix 1

University of Wales College of Medicine
School of Nursing Studies
Heath Park, Cardiff

Nurse Education and Experiential Learning Questionnaire

I am interested in your views on nurse education and experiential
learning. Experiential learning and experiential learning methods
have been defined in various ways and this questionnaire has been
developed from a number of nurse tutors' and student nurses' views
about learning from experience.

This questionnaire has **THREE** parts. Please fill in each part.

In Part **ONE** you are asked about experiential learning methods.

In Part **TWO** you are asked about your views on nurse education and
experiential learning.

In Part **THREE** you are asked for brief details about yourself.

249

The questionnaire will take you about 15 minutes to complete. Do not spend too long on each item but make sure that you answer each one. There are no right or wrong answers and your replies will be treated in confidence.

Thank you for your cooperation in this study.

Philip Burnard,
Lecturer in Nursing Studies,
School of Nursing Studies,
University of Wales College of Medicine,
Heath Park, Cardiff.

PART ONE

Experiential learning methods

In this section, please put a tick against any of the experiential learning methods that you have used or taken part in as part of a nurse education programme. You may tick as many or as few items as appropriate.

Icebreaker activities

Role-Play

Psychodrama

Small group discussion

Simulations

Practising clinical nursing skills

Exercises that involve reflection on past or present experience

Empathy building exercises

Problem solving exercises

The "blind walk" exercise

Structured group activities

Transactional analysis exercises

Gestalt exercises

Please list below any OTHER experiential learning activities that
you have taken part in or used.

_____

_____

_____

_____

_____

PART TWO

In this section, you are offered a series of statements about aspects
of nurse education and experiential learning. Next to each
statement, please circle one of the following, to indicate how you
feel about the statement :

SA   A   U   D   SD

(Strongly Agree) (Agree) (Uncertain) (Disagree) (Strongly Disagree)

Your perceptions of nurse education

1. Student nurses are allowed to negotiate their learning
programme with their tutors.
SA   A   U   D   SD

2. Student nurses learn most about nursing in the school of nursing.
SA   A   U   D   SD

3. Student nurses learn best from personal experience.
SA   A   U   D   SD

4. "School" learning and "clinical" learning are not always linked.

SA   A   U   D   SD

5. Students are free to choose the learning method that suits them best.
SA   A   U   D   SD

6. Students learn most about nursing in the clinical situation.
SA   A   U   D   SD

7. Students learn most about nursing by observing other nurses at work.
SA   A   U   D   SD

Definitions of Experiential Learning

1. Experiential learning is learning that takes place in the clinical setting.
SA   A   U   D   SD

2. Experiential learning is learning from life experience.
SA   A   U   D   SD

3. Experiential learning is not "textbook" learning.
SA   A   U   D   SD

4. Experiential learning is "practical" learning rather than "theoretical" learning.
SA   A   U   D   SD

5. Experiential learning can be a form of therapy for students.
SA   A   U   D   SD

6. Experiential learning does not involve lectures.
SA   A   U   D   SD

7. Experiential learning is learning by doing.
SA   A   U   D   SD

8. Experiential learning can be a form of therapy for tutors.
SA   A   U   D   SD

9. Experiential learning is difficult to define.
SA   A   U   D   SD

10. Experiential learning is concerned with learning more about how you feel.
SA   A   U   D   SD

Experiential Learning Methods in Action

1. Experiential learning methods are useful for learning interpersonal skills.
SA   A   U   D   SD

2. Experiential learning methods are easy to take part in.
SA   A   U   D   SD

3. Experiential learning methods encourage you to reflect on your nursing practice.
SA   A   U   D   SD

4. Experiential learning methods are easier to use than other learning methods.
SA   A   U   D   SD

5. Experiential learning methods do not suit all students.
SA   A   U   D   SD

6. Experiential learning methods can be fun.
SA   A   U   D   SD

7. Experiential learning methods are the best methods for learning about nursing.
SA   A   U   D   SD

8. Experiential learning methods can feel unrealistic.
SA   A   U   D   SD

9. Experiential learning methods can increase self-awareness.
SA   A   U   D   SD

10. Experiential learning methods suit all teachers.
SA   A   U   D   SD

11. Experiential learning methods can be embarrassing.
SA   A   U   D   SD

12. Experiential learning methods are suitable for learning all aspects of nursing.
SA   A   U   D   SD

13. Experiential learning methods can be used in the clinical setting.
SA   A   U   D   SD

14. Experiential learning methods used in the school are useful for learning about nursing.
SA   A   U   D   SD

15. I don't like experiential learning methods.
SA   A   U   D   SD

16. Experiential learning methods can be time consuming.
SA   A   U   D   SD

17. Experiential learning methods help students to learn practical nursing skills.
SA   A   U   D   SD

18. I prefer experiential learning methods to other learning methods.
SA   A   U   D   SD

19. Experiential learning sessions could get out of control.
SA   A   U   D   SD

PART THREE

1. Your job : Tick one of the following:

Nurse Educator

Student Nurse

2. Your Gender : Tick one of the following:

Female

Male

3. Your Age : Tick one of the following:

18 - 21

22 - 30

31 - 40

41 - 50

Over 50

3. Your <u>main</u> area of work or study : Tick one of the following:

General Nursing

Psychiatric Nursing

Mental Handicap
Nursing

Thank you for filling in this questionnaire : Philip Burnard 1990

Appendix 2

OTHER EXPERIENTIAL LEARNING METHODS IDENTIFIED FROM
QUESTIONNAIRES

This is a list of methods that questionnaire respondents identified in
the section marked "Please list below any other experiential
learning activities that you have taken part in or used."

Clinical activities

Community observation
Aseptic technique
Observation visits to different care settings
Visits to other institutions
Teaching "on the job"
Trial and error learning

Classroom activities

Guided study
Board games
Flipcharts
Group projects
Library research

Communications exercises
Planning teaching exercises
Teaching of skills
Brainstorming
Management training
Decision making
Project presentation
Contract learning
Lecturing

Use of technology

Computer simulations
Videos
Video taped patient interaction
Computer aided learning
Films
Audio-taped exercises

Self-Awareness/Therapy Activities

Stress relieving exercises
Guided phantasy
Group sculptures
Survival training
Shop Mobility : spending time in a city centre in a wheelchair
Trust exercises
Neurolinguistic programming exercises
Outdoor pursuits
Group analysis
Spontaneous drawing
Counselling workshops
Self-awareness exercises
Family therapy

References

A.A.H.P. 1962 *Articles of Association* : Association for Humanistic Psychology : San Francisco, California.

Abrahams, P. 1984 Evaluating Soft Findings : Some Problems of Measuring Informal Care : *Research, Policy and Planning* : 2 : 2 : 1 - 8.

Adler, A. 1927 *The Practice and Theory of Individual Psychology* : Harcourt, Brace, Jovanovitch, New York.

Alberti, R.E. and Emmons, M.L. 1982 *Your Perfect Right : a Guide to Assertive Living* : Impact, San Luis Obispo, California.

Alexander, M.F. 1983 *Learning to Nurse : Integrating Theory and Practice* : Churchill Livingstone, Edinburgh.

Altschul, A. 1972 *Patient-Nurse Interaction* : Churchill Livingston, Edinburgh.

Anderson, H.H. (ed) 1959 *Creativity and Its Cultivation* : Harper and Row, New York.

Argyle, M. 1975 *The Psychology of Interpersonal Behaviour* : Penguin, Harmondsworth.

Argyle, M. 1981 *Social Skills and Work* : Methuen, London.

Arnold, E. and Boggs, K. 1989 *Interpersonal Relations : Professional Communication Skills for Nurses* : Saunders, Philadelphia.

Aronson, E. 1980 *The Social Animal* : 3rd Edition : Freeman, San Francisco.

Ashton, J. and Seymour, H. 1988 *The New Public Health* : Open University Press, Milton Keynes.

Atkinson, R.L., Atkinson, R.C., Smith, E.E., Bem, D.J. and Hilgard, E.R. 1990 *Introduction to Psychology* : 10th Edition : Harcourt Brace Jovanovich, Orlando, Florida.

Babbie, E. 1979 *The Practice of Social Research* : 3rd edition : Wadsworth, Belmont, California.

Back, K.W. 1972 *Beyond Words : The Story of Sensitivity Training and the Encounter Movement* : Russell Sage, New York.

Bailey, C.R. 1983 Experiential Learning and the Curriculum : *Nursing Times* : July 20th : 45 - 46.

Ball, S.J. 1984 Beachside Reconsidered : Reflections on a Methodological Apprenticeship. In R.G. Burgess (ed) *The Research Process in Educational Settings : Ten Case Studies* : Falmer Press, London.

Bandler, R. and Grinder, J. 1975 *The Structure of Magic* : Vol I : Science and Behaviour Books, California

Bandler, R. and Grinder, J. 1979 *Frogs into Princes : Neurolinguistic Programming* : Real People Press, Moab, Utah.

Bandler, R. and Grinder, J. 1982 *Reframing : Neurolinguistic Programming and the Transformation of Meaning* : Real People Press, Moab, Utah.

Bannister, D. and Fransella, F. 1986 *Inquiring Man : The Psychology of Personal Constructs* : 3rd Edition : Croom Helm, London.

Barber, P. and Norman, I. 1987 Skills in Supervision : *Nursing Times* : 83 : 14th January : 56 - 57.

Barnes, D.M. 1983 Teaching Communication Skills to Student Nurses - an Experience : *Nurse Education Today* : 13 : 2 : 45 - 48.

Barrell, J.J., Mederiros, D. and Barrell, J.E. 1985 The Causes and Treatment of Performance Anxiety : An

Experiential Approach : *Journal of Humanistic Psychology* : 25 : 2 : 106 - 122.

Barron, M.E. and Krulee, G.K. 1948 Case Study of a Basic Skill Training Group. Reprinted in T.L. Harris and W.E. Schwahn, W.E. 1961 *Selected Readings on the Learning Process* : Oxford University Press, New York.

Berg, B.L. 1989 *Qualitative Research Methods for the Social Sciences* : Allyn and Bacon, New York.

Bernstein, B. 1972 Social Class, Language and Socialisation. In P.P. Giglioli. *Language and Social Context* : Penguin, Harmondsworth.

Blatner, A. 1988 *Foundations of Psychodrama : History, Theory and Practice* : 3rd Edition : Springer, London.

Bloor, M. 1978 On the Analysis of Observational Data. In Berg, B.L. 1989 *Qualitative Research Methods for the Social Sciences* : Allyn and Bacon, New York.

Bogdan, R.C. and Biklen, S.K. 1982 *Qualitative Research for Education : An Introduction to Theory and Practice* :Wiley, Chichester.

Bond, M. 1986 *Stress and Self-Awareness : A Guide for Nurses* : Heinemann, London.

Bond, M. and Kilty, J. 1983 *Practical Ways of Coping With Stress* : Human Potential Research Project : University of Surrey, Guildford, Surrey.

Bond, S. 1990 Primary Nursing and Primary Medical Care : *Nursing Times* : 86 : 25 : 57.

Boud, D., Keogh, R. and Walker, D. 1985 *Reflection : Turning Experience into Learning* : Kogan Page, London.

Boud, D. and Pascoe, J. 1978 *Experiential Learning : Developments in Australian Post-Secondary Education* : Australian Consortium on Experiential Education, Sydney, Australia.

Boudieu, P. 1971 Systems of Education and Systems of Thought. In M.F.D. Young : *Knowledge and Control : New Directions for the Sociology of Education* : Collier Macmillan, London.

Bowen, D. 1990 *Shaking the Iron Universe* : Hodder and Stoughton : London.

Boydell, T. 1976 *Experiential Learning* : Manchester Monograph No. 5 : Universtity of Manchester, Manchester.

Bracken, E. and Davis, J. 1989 The Implications of Mentorship in Nursing Career Development : *Senior Nurse* : 9 : 15 - 16.

Brande, D. 1981 *Becoming a Writer* : Macmillan, London.

Brookfield, S.D. 1986 *Understanding and Facilitating Adult Learning : A Comprehensive Analysis of Principles and Effective Practices* : Open University Press, Milton Keynes.

Brookfield, S. D.1987 *Developing Critical Thinkers : Challenging Adults to Explore Alternative Ways of Thinking and Acting* :Open University Press, Milton Keynes.

Bryman, A. 1988 *Quantity and Quality in Social Research* : Allan and Unwin, London.

Bullock, A. and Stallybrass, O. 1977 *The Fontana Dictionary of Modern Thought* : Fontana/Collins, London.

Burnard, P. 1983 Through Experience and From Experience : *Nursing Mirror* : 156 : 9 : 29 - 33.

Burnard, P. 1984 Paradigms for Progress : *Senior Nurse* : 1 : 38 : 24 - 26.

Burnard, P. 1985 *Learning Human Skills ; a Guide for Nurses* : Heinemann, London.

Burnard, P. 1986 Encountering Adults : *Senior Nurse* : 4 : 4 : 30 - 31.

Burnard, P. 1987a Towards an Epistemological Basis for Experiential Learning : *Journal of Advanced Nursing* : 12 : 189 - 193.

Burnard, P. 1987b *A Study of the Ways in Which Experiential Learning Methods Are Used to Develop Interpersonal Skills in Nurses in Canada and the United States of America* : Florence Nightingale Memorial Committee, London.

Burnard, P. 1988a Experiential Learning : Some Theoretical Considerations : *International Journal of Lifelong Education* : 7 : 2 : 127 - 133.

Burnard, P. 1988b Experiential Learning : Some Theoretical Considerations : *International Journal of Lifelong Education* : 7 : 2 : 127 - 133.

Burnard, P. 1988c The Journal as an Assessment and Evaluation Tool in Nurse Education : *Nurse Education Today* : 8 : 105 - 107.

Burnard, P. 1989a Experiential Learning and Andragogy - Negotiated Learning in Nurse Education : a Critical Appraisal : *Nurse Education Today* : 9 : 5 : 300 - 306.

Burnard, P. 1989b Exploring Nurse Educators' Views of Experiential Learning : a Pilot Study : *Nurse Education Today* : 9 : 1 : 39 -45.

Burnard, P. 1989c *Teaching Interpersonal Skills : A Handbook of Experiential Learning for Health Professionals* : Chapman and Hall, London.

Burnard, P. 1990d *Counselling Skills for Health Professionals* : Chapman and Hall, London.

Burnard, P. 1990 *Learning Human Skills : An Experiential Guide for Nurses* : 2nd Edition : Heinemann, Oxford.

Burnard, P. and Chapman, C.M. 1988 *Professional and EthicalIssues in Nursing : The Code of Professional Conduct* : Wiley,Chichester.

Butterworth, T. 1984 The Future Training of Psychiatric and General Nurses : *Nursing Times* : July 25th : 65 - 66.

Carney, J. 1982 *Content Analysis* : Harper and Row, London.

Carper, B.A. 1978 Fundamental Patterns of Knowing in Nursing : *Advances in Nursing Science* : 1 : 1 : 13 - 23.

Caxton, G. 1984 *Live and Learn : An Introduction to the Psychology of Growth and Change in Everyday Life* : Harper and Row, London.

Clare, A. with Thompson, S. 1981 *Let's Talk About Me!* : BBC, London.

Clarke, M. 1986 Action and Reflection : Practice and Theory in Nursing : *Journal of Advanced Nursing* : 11 : 3 - 11.

Clark, D.H. and Kadis, A.L. 1971 *Humanistic Teaching* : Merrill, Columbus, Ohio.

Clarke, B. and Feltham, W. 1990 Facilitating Peer Group Teaching Within Nurse Education : *Nurse Education Today* : 10 : 54 - 57.

Clift, J.C. and Imrie, B.W. 1981 *Assessing Students and Apprasing Teaching* : Croom Helm, London.

Cook, T. and Reichardt, C. (eds) 1979 *Qualitative and Quantative Methods in Evaulation Research* : Sage, Beverly Hills, California.

Cormack, D. 1976 *Psychiatric Nursing Observed* : RCN, London.

Costello, J. 1989 Learning From Each Other : Peer Teaching and Learning In Student Nurse Training : *Nurse Education Today* : 9 : 203 - 206.

Couchman, W. and Dawson, J. 1990 *Nursing and Health -Care Research : The Use and Applications of Research for Nurses and Other Health Care Professionals* : Scutari, London.

Cox, M. 1978 *Structuring the Therapuetic Process* : Pergamon, London.

Degerando, J. 1800 [1969] *Considerations on the Various Methods to Follow in the Observation of Savage People* (Trans F.C.T. Moore) University of California, Berkeley.

Dewey, J. 1916 *Democracy and Education* : Free Press,London.

Dewey, J. 1933 *How We Think* : D.C. Heath, Boston.

Dewey, J. 1938 *Experience and Education* : Collier Macmillan, London.

Dietrich, G.C. 1978 Teaching of Psychiatric Nursing in the Classroom : *Journal of Advanced Nursing* : 3 : 525 - 534.

Dillman, D.A. 1978 *Mail and Telephone Surveys* : Wiley, New York

Donovan, J. 1990 The Concept and Role of Mentor : *Nurse Education Today* : 10 : 294 - 298.

Douglas, J. 1985 *Investigative Social Research* : Sage, Beverly Hills, California

Dowd, C. 1983 Learning Through Experience : *Nursing Times* : 7th July : 50 - 52.

Dubin, S. and Okun, M. 1973 Implications of Learning Theories for Adult Instruction : *Adult Education* : 24 : 1 : 3 - 19.

Dux, C.M. 1989 An Investigation Into Whether Nurse Teachers Take Into Account the Individual Learning

Styles of the Students When Formulating Teaching Strategies : *Nurse Education Today* : 9 : 186 - 191.

Egan, G. 1977 *You and Me* : Brooks/Cole, Monterey, California.

Egan, G. 1990 *The Skilled Helper* : 4th Edition : Brooks/Cole, Pacific Grove, California.

Ellis, R. and Watson, C. 1987 Experiential Learning : The Development of Communication Skills in a Group Therapy Setting : *Journal of Advanced Nursing* : 7 : 215 - 221.

Ellis, R. and Whittington, D. 1981 *A Guide to Social Skills Training* : Croom Helm, London.

ENB 1982 *Syllabus of Training : Professional Register - Part 3 : (Registered Mental Nurse* : English National Board for Nursing, Midwifery and Health Visiting, London

END 1987 *Managing Change in Nurse Education* : English National Board for Nursing, Midwifery and Health Visting, London.

Epting, F. 1984 *Personal Construct Counselling and Psychothorupy* : Wiley, Chichester.

F.E.U. 1983 *Curriculum Opportunity : A Map of Experiential Learning in Entry Requirements to Higher and further Education Award Bearing Courses* : Further Education Unit, London.

Field, P.A. and Morse, J.M. 1985 *Nursing Research : The Application of Qualitative Approaches* : Croom Helm, London.

Fielding, P. 1983 *An Evaluation of Videotaping Teaching Material* : Unpublished report : King Edward's Hospital Fund, London.

Filstead, W.J. 1970 Qualitative Methods : A Needed Perspective in Evaluation Research. In T.Cook and C. Reichardt (eds) *Qualitatitive and Quantative Methods in Evaluation Research* : Sage, Beverly Hills, California.

Fink, A and Kosekoff, J. 1985 *How to Conduct Surveys : A step-by-step guide* : Sage, Beverly Hills, California

Fox, D.J. 1982 *Fundamentals of Research in Nursing* : 4th Edition : Appleton-Century-Crofts, Norwalk, New Jersey.

265

Fox, R. 1975 *Encounter With Anthropology* : Peregrine, Harmondsworth.

Freire, P. 1972 *Pedagogy of the Oppressed* : Penguin, Harmondsworth.

Fretwell, J.E. 1982 *Ward Teaching and Learning* : RCN, London.

Fromm, E. 1957 *The Art of Loving* : Unwin, London

Fromm 1979 *To Have or to Be?* : Abacus Books, London

Garratt, R. 1983 The Power of Action Learning. In M. Pedlar :(ed) *Action Learning in Practice* : Gower, Aldershot.

Gaut, D. 1984 A Philosophic Orientation to Caring Research. In M. Leninger (ed) Care : *The Essence of Nursing and Health* : Slack, Thorofare, New Jersey.

Getzels, J.W. and Jackson, P.W. 1962 *Creativity and Intelligence* : Wiley, Chichester.

Ginsburg, C. 1984 Towards a Somatic Understanding of Self : *Journal of Humanistic Psychology* : 24 : 2 : 66 - 92.

Gladstone, G. 1990 Bioenergetics and Psychodrama at the Open Centre : *Self and Society : The European Journal of Humanistic Psychology* : XVIII:3:28 - 31.

Glaser, B.G. and Strauss, A.L. 1967 *The Discovery of Grounded Theory* : Aldine, New York.

Goble, J. 1990 Psychodrama Takes Centre Stage : *Nursing Times* : 86 : 28 : 34 - 35.

Goffman, E. 1961 *Asylums* : Penguin, Harmondsworth.

Gonen, J.Y. 1971 The Use of Psychodrama combined with Videotaped Playback on an In-Patient Floor : *Psychiatry* : 34 : 198 - 213.

Gott, M. 1984 *Learning Nursing* : RCN, London.

Grossman, R. 1985 Some Reflections on Abraham Maslow : *Journal of Humanistic Psychology* : 25 : 4 : 31 -34.

Grundy, S. 1982 Three Modes of Action Research : *Curriculum Perspectives* : 2 : 3 : 136 - 142.

Hall, C. 1984 *A Primer of Freudian Psychology* : Mentor Books, New York.

Hamilton, D. 1986 *Curriculum Evaluation* : Open Books, London.

Hampden-Turner, C. 1966 An Existential Learning Theory : *Journal of Applied Behavioural Science* : 12 : 4 : 36 - 43.

Harvey, T.J. and Vaughan J. 1990 Student Nurse Attitudes Towards Different Teaching/Learning Methods : *Nurse Education Today* : 10 : 181 - 185.

Heath, J. 1983 Gaming/Simulation in Nurse Education : *Nurse Education Today* : 13 : 4 : 92 - 95.

Heidegger, M. 1927 *Being and Time* : Harper and Row, New York.

Henry, J. 1989 Meaning and Practice in Experiential Learning. In S.W. Weil and I. McGill *Making Sense of Experiential Learning : Diversity in Theory and Practice* : Open University Press, Milton Keynes.

Heron, J. 1973 *Experiential Training Techniques* : Human Potential Research Project, University of Surrey, Guildford.

Heron, J. 1975 *Experience and Method* : Human Potential Research Project : University of Surrey, Guildford.

Heron, J. 1977a *Catharsis in Human Development* : Human Potential Research Project, University of Surrey, Guildford.

Heron, J. 1977b *Behaviour Analysis in Education and Training* : Human Potential Research Project : University of Surrey, Guildford.

Heron, J. 1978 *Co-Counselling Teachers Manual* : Human Potential Research Project, University of Surrey, Guildford.

Heron, J. 1981 Philosophical Basis for a New Paradigm. In P. Reason and J. Rowan (eds) *Human Inquiry : A sourcebook of new paradigm research* : Wiley, Chichester.

Heron, J. 1982 *Experiential Training Techniques* : 2nd Edition : Human Potential Resouce Group : University of Surrey, Guildford.

Heron J. 1983 *Education of the Affect*: Human Potential Research Project, University of Surrey, Guildford.

Heron, J. 1989a *The Facilitators' Handbook* : Kogan Page, London

Heron, J. 1989b *Six Category Intervention Analysis* : 3rd Edition :Human Potential Resource Group : University of Surrey, Guildford.

Hinkle, D. 1965 *The Change of Personal Constructs from the Viewpoint of a Theory of Construct Implications* : PhD thesis : Ohio State University, Ohio.

Hirst, P.H. 1972 Liberal Education and the Nature of Knowledge. In R.D. Archambault (ed) : *Philosophical Analysis and Education* : Routeldge and Kegan Paul, London.

Hirst, P. and Peters, R.S. 1970 *The Logic of Education* : Routledge and Kegan Paul, London.

HMSO 1944 *Education Act* : HMSO, London

Holt, J. 1964 *How Children Fail* : Penguin, Harmondsworth.

Horney, K. 1937 *The Neurotic Personality of Our Time* : Norton, New York.

Howard, A. 1990 Counselling PLC : *Counselling : The Journal of the British Association for Counselling* : 1 : 1 : 15 - 16.

Hudson, K. 1983 *The Dictionary of the Teenage Revolution and its Aftermath* : Macmillan, London.

Huges, G. 1988 *Words in Time : A Social History of the English Vocabulary* : Blackwell, Oxford.

Hugh-Jones, P., Tanser, A. and Whitby, C. 1964 Patients' View of Admission to a London Teaching Hospital : *British Medical Journal* : 9 : 660 -664.

Husserl, E. 1931 Ideas : *General Introduction to Pure Phenomenology* : trans G. Boyce : Allen and Unwin, London.

Iwasiw, C.L. and Sleightholm - Cairns, B. 1990 Clinical Conferences - the Key to Successful Experiential Learning : *Nurse Education Today* : 10 : 260 - 265.

James, W. 1902 *The Varieties of Religious Experience* : Random House, Toronto.

James, W.B. 1983 *An Analysis of Perceptions of the Practices of Adult Educators From Five Different Settings* : Proceedings of theAdult Education Research Conference, No. 24 : Concordia University/ University of Montreal, Canada.

Jarvis, P. 1983 *Professional Education* : Croom Helm, London.

Jarvis, P. 1984 *The Theory and Practice of Adult and Continuing Education* : Croom Helm, London

Jarvis, P. 1987 *Adult Learning in the Social Context* : Croom Helm, London.

Jarvis, P. and Gibson, S. 1985 *The Teacher Practitioner in Nursing, Midwifery and Health Visiting* : Croom Helm, London.

Jasmin, S. and Hill, L. 1978 Videotaping and Interpersonal Skills Development : *Nursing Leadership* : 1 : 4 - 10.

Jones, R.G. 1990 The Lecture as a Teaching Method in Modern Nurse Education : *Nurse Education Today* : 10 : 290 - 293.

Jourard, S. 1964 *The Transparent Self* : Van Nostrand, Princeton,New Jersey.

Jones, D. 1990 Editorial : *Self and Society : The European Journal of Humanistic Psychology* : XVIII : 3 : 1.

Jung, C.G. 1931 *Modern Man In Search of a Soul* : Rascher, Zurich.

Kagan, C.M. (ed) 1985 *Interpersonal Skills in Nursing : Research and Applications* : Croom Helm, London.

Kagan, C., Evans, J. and Kay, B. 1986 *A Manual of Interpersonal Skills for Nurses : An Experiential Approach* : Harper and Row, London.

Kalisch, B.J. 1971 Strategies for Developing Nurses Empathy : *Nursing Outlook* : 19 : 11 : 714 - 717.

Keeton, M. and Associates 1976 *Experiential Learning* : Jossey Bass, San Francisco, California,

Kelly, G. 1955 *The Psychology of Personal Constructs* : Volumes 1 and 2 : Norton, New York.

Kelly, V. 1977 *The Curriculum* : Harper and Row, London

Kenworthy, N. and Nicklin, P. 1989 *Teaching and Assessing in Nursing Practice* : Scutari, London.

Kidd, J.R. 1973 *How Adults Learn* : Cambridge Books, New York.

Kidder, L.H. and Judd, M. 1986 *Research Methods in Social Relations* : CBS Publishing, Japan.

Kilty, J. 1983 *Experiential Learning* : Human Potential Research Project, University of Surrey, Guildford.

Kilty, J. 1984 *Self and Peer Assessment* : Human Potential Research Project, University of Surrey, Guildford.

Kirschenbaum, H. 1979 *On Becoming Carl Rogers* : Dell, New York.

Knowles, M.S. 1978 *The Adult Learner : A Neglected Species* : 2nd Edition : Gulf, Texas.

Knowles, M.S. 1980 *The Modern Practice of Adult Education : From Pedaggoy to Andragogy* :2nd Edition : Follett, Chicago.

Knowles M. S. and Associates 1984 *Andragogy in Action :Applying Modern Principles of Adult Learning* : Jossey Bass,San Francisco, California.

Kolb, D. 1984 *Experiential Learning* : Prentice Hall, Englewood Cliffs, New York

Kopp, S. 1972 *If You Meet the Buddha on the Road, Kill Him. A modern pilgramage through myth, legend, zen and psychotherapy* : Sheldon Press, London.

Langford, M.J. 1990 The Moot Court in Teaching Bioethics : *Nurse Education Today* :10 : 24 - 30.

Lasker, H, Moore, J. and Simpson, E.L. 1980 *Adult Development and Approaches to Learning* : National Institute of Education, Washington, DC.

Lawton, D. 1973 *Social Change, Educational Theory and Curriculum Planning* : Hodder and Stoughton, London

Leininger, M.M. (ed) 1985 *Qualiatative Research Methods in Nursing* : Grune and Stratton, New York.

Lewin, K. 1952 *Field Theory and Social Change* : Tavistock, London.

Ley, P. 1972 Complaints Made By Hospital Staff and Patients : a Review of the Literature : *Bulletin of British Psychological Society* : 25 : 115 - 120.

Lieberman, M.A., Yalom, I.D. and Miles, M.B. 1973 *Encounter Groups : First Facts* : Basic Books, New York.

Lipton, L. 1960 *The Holy Barbairans* : W.H. Allen, New York.

Lofland, J. 1971 *Analysing Social Settings : a Guide to Qualitative Observation and Analysis* : Wadsworth, Belmont, California.

Logan, J.C. 1971 Use of Psychodrama and Sociodrama in Reducing Negro Agression : *Group Psychotherapy and Psychodrama* : 24 : 138 - 149.

Luft, J. 1967 *Of Human Interaction : The Johari Model* : Mayfield, Palo Alto, California.

Lyte, V.J. and Thompson, I.G. 1990 The Diary as a Formative Teaching and Learning Aid Incorporating Means of

Evaluating and Renegotiation of Clinical Learning
Objectives : *Nurse Education Today* : 10 : 228 - 232.

Mackay, R. and Carver, R. (eds) 1990 *Empathy in the Helping
Relationship* : Springer, New York.

Macleod-Clark, J. 1985 The Development of Research in
Interpersonal Skills in Nursing. In C.Kagan (ed)
*Interpersonal Skills in Nursing : Research and
Applications* : Croom Helm, London,

Macquarrie, J. 1972 *Existentialism* : Penquin,
Harmondsworth,

Mahrer, A.L. 1989 A Case of Fundamentally Different
Existential-Humanistic Psychologies : *Journal of
Humanistic Psychology* : 29 : 2 : 249 - 261.

Main, A. 1985 Reflection and the Development of Learning
Skills. In D. Boud, R. Keogh and D. Walker. 1985
Reflection : Turning Experience into Learning : Kogan
Page, London.

Marshfield, G. 1985 Issues Arising from Teaching
Interpersonal Skills in General Nurse Training. In C.
Kagan (ed) *Interpersonal Skills in Nursing : Research
and Applications* : Croom Helm, London.

Marson, S.N. 1979 Nursing : a Helping Relationship? :
Nursing Times : March 29th : 541 - 544.

Maslow, A. 1972 *Motivation and Personality* : 2nd Edition :
Harper and Row, London.

Masson, J. 1990 *Against Therapy* : Fontana, London.

May, R. 1989 Answer to Ken Wilber and John Rowan :
Journal of Humanistic Psychology : 29 : 2 : 244 - 248.

McGhee, A. 1961 *The Patients' Attitude to Nursing Care* :
Churchill Livingstone, Edinburgh.

McNulty, M. 1984 A Framework for the Future : *Nursing
Mirror* : 158 :9 : pages not numbered.

Mella, K. 1986 *Learning and Working* : Churchill
Livingstone, Edinburgh.

Meziro, J. 1981 A Critical Theory of Adult Learning and
Education : *Adult Education* : 32 : 1 : 3 - 24.

Miles, R. 1987 Experiential Learning in the Classroom. In P.
Allen and M. Jolley (eds) *The Curriculum in Nursing
education* : Croom Helm, London.

Milne, D., Burdett, C. and Beckett, J. 1986 Assessing and Reducing the Stress and Strain of Psychiatric Nursing : *Nursing Times* : 82 : 19 : 59 - 62.

Minton, D. 1984 Evaluation and Assessment in Continuing Education. In *Teaching Strategies for Continuing Education* : City and Guilds Institute, London.

Moreno, J.L. 1959 *Psychodrama* : Volume two : Beacon House Press, Beacon, New York.

Moreno, J.L. 1969 *Psychodrama* : Volume three : Beacon House Press, Beacon, New York.

Moreno, J.L. 1977 *Psychodrama* : Volume one : 4th Edition : Beacon House Press, Beacon, New York.

Moser, J.A. and Kalton, G. 1971 *Survey Methods in Social Investigation* : Heinemann, London.

Murgatroyd, S. 1986 *Counselling and Helping* : Methuen, London.

Murgatroyd, S. and Woolfe, R. 1982 *Coping With Crisis : Understanding and Helping People in Need* : Harper and Row, London.

Murphy, G. and Kovach, J.K. 1972 *Historical Introduction to Modern Psychology* : 6th Edition : Routledge and Kegan Paul, London.

Nelson-Jones, R. 1981 *The Theory and Practice of Counselling Psychology* : Holt, Rhinehart and Winston, London.

Nieswiadomy, R.M. 1987 *Foundations of Nursing Research* : Appleton and Lange, Norwalk, Connecticut.

Norton, D, McLaren, R. and Exton-Smith, A. 1976 *An Investigation of Geriatric Nursing Problems in Hospital* : Churchill Livingston, Edinburgh.

Nye, R.D. 1986 *Three Psychologies : Perspectives from Freud, Skinner and Rogers* : 3rd Edition : Brooks/cole, Monterey, California.

O'Kell, S.P. 1988 A Study of the Relationships Between Learning Style, Readiness for Self-Directed learning and Teaching Preference of Learner Nurses in One Health District : *Nurse Education Today* : 8 : 197 - 204.

Ogier, M.E. 1982 *An Ideal Sister* : RCN, London.

Oiler, C. 1982 The Phenomenological Approach in Nursing Research : *Nursing research* : 31 : 178-181

Oppenheim, A.N. 1966 *Questionnaire Design and Attitude Measurement* : Heinemann, London.

Orton, H.D. 1981 *Ward Learning Climate* : RCN, London.

Palmer, R. and Pope, C. 1984 *Brain Train : Studying for Success* : Spon, London.

Pankhurst, R. 1987 In and Out of the Stream : *Self and Society : The European Journal of Humanistic Psychology* : XV : 3 : 134 - 138.

Parlett, M. 1981 Illuminative Evaluation. In P. Reason and J. Rowan (eds) *Human Inquiry : A Sourcebook of New Paradigm Research* : Wiley, Chichester.

Patka, F. (ed) 1972 *Existential Thinkers and Thought* : Citadel, Secaucus, New Jersey.

Patton, M.Q. 1982 *Practical Evaluation* : Sage, Beverly Hills, California.

Pedler, M. (ed) 1983 *Action Learning in Practice* : Gower, Aldershot.

Pelto, P. 1970 *Anthropological Research : The Structure of Inquiry* : Harper and Row, New York.

Perls, F. 1973 *The Gestalt Approach and Eyewitness to Therapy* : Science and Behaviour Books, Palo Alto, California.

Perry, L.R. 1972 What is an Educational Situation? In R.D. Archambault (ed) : *Philosophical Analysis and Education* : Routledge and Kegan Paul, London.

Peters, R.S. 1966 *Ethics and Education* : Allen and Unwin, London.

Peters, R.S. 1972 *Education as Initiation*. In R.D. Archambault(ed) Philosophical Analysis and Education : Routledge and Kegan Paul, London.

Pfeiffer, J.W. and Goodstein, L.D. 1982 *The 1982 Annual for Facilitators, Trainers and Consultants* : University Associates, San Diego, California.

Pfeiffer, J.W. and Jones, J.E. 1974 *A Handbook of Structured Experiences for Human Relations Training* : Vol 1 : University Associates, La Jolla, California.

Pilcher, D.M. 1990 *Data Analysis for the Helping Professions : A Practical Guide* : Sage, Newbury Park, California.

Polanyi, M. 1958 *Personal Knowledge* : University of Chicago Press, Chicago.

Pollock, L.C. 1989 *Community Psychiatric Nursing : Myth and Reality* : Scutari, London

Porritt, L. 1990 *Interaction Strategies : an Introduction for Health Professionals* : 2nd Edition : Churchill Livingstone, Edinburgh.

Postman, N. and Weingartner, C. 1969 *Teaching as a Subversive Activity* : Penguin, Harmondsworth.

Postuma, A.B. and Postuma, B.W.1973 *Some Observations of Encounter Casualties* : Journal of Applied Behavioural Sciences : 9 : 595 - 608.

Powell, J.P. 1985 Autobiographical Learning. In D. Boud, R. Keogh and D. Walker. 1985 *Reflection : Turning Experience into Learning* : Kogan Page, London.

Price, D.D. and Barrell, J.J. 1980 An Experiential Approach With Quantitative Methods : A Research Paradigm : *Journal of Humanistic Psychology* : 20 : 3 : 75 - 95.

Pring, R. 1976 *Knowledge and Schooling* : Basic Books, London.

Quinsland, L.K. and Van Ginkel, A. 1984 How to Process Experience : *Journal of Experiential Education* : 7 : 2 : 8 - 13.

Raggucci, A.T. 1972 The Ethnographic Approach and Nursing Research : *Nursing Research* : 21 : 485 - 490.

Raichura, L. 1987 Learning by Doing : *Nursing Times* : 83 : 13 : 59 - 61.

Reason, P. and Rowan, J. 1981 *Human Inquiry : A Sourcebook of New Paradigm Research* : Wiley, Chichester.

Reed, E.J. 1984 Using Psychodrama With Critical Care Nurses : *Dimensions of Critical Care Nursing* : 3 : 2 : 110 - 114.

Reilly, D.E. and Oermann, M.H. 1985 *The Clinical Field : Its Use in Nursing Education* : Appleton-Century-Crofts, Norwalk, Connecticut.

Revans, R.W. 1978 *The ABC of Action Learning : a Review of 25 Years of Experience* : Action Learning Trust, Luton.

Revans, R.W. 1982 *The Origins and Growth of Action Learning* : Chartwell-Bratt, Bickley, Kent.

Reyner, J.H. 1984 *The Gurdjieff Inheritance* : Turnstone Press, Wellinborough.

274

Reynold, W. 1985 Issues Arising From Teaching Interpersonal
Skills in Psychiatric Nurse Training. In C. Kagan, (ed).
*Interpersonal Skills in Nursing : Research and
Applications* : Croom Helm, London.

Reynolds, W. and Cormack, D. 1987 Teaching Psychiatric
Nursing : Interpersonal Skills. In B. Davis : *Nurse
Education : Research and Developments* : Croom
Helm, London.

Richardson, M., Bishop, J., Caygill, D., Mace, C., Ross, R,
Taylor, S. and Tuczemskyi, E. 1990 : Disabled for a
Day : *Nursing Times* : 86 : 21 : 66 - 67.

Riehl-Sisca, J. 1989 *Conceptual Models for Nursing
Practice* : Appleton and Lange, New York.

Rogers, C.R. 1952 *Client Centred Therapy* : Constable,
London.

Rogers, C.R. 1957 The Necessary and Sufficient Conditions
of Therapuetic Personality Change : *Journal of
Consulting Psychology* : 21 : 95-104.

Rogers, C.R. 1967 *On Becoming a Person* : Constable,
London

Rogers, C.R. 1970 *On Encounter Groups* : Penguin,
Harmondsworth

Rogers, C.R. 1972 The Facilitation of Significant Learning.
In M.L. Silberman, J.S. Allender and J.M. Yanoff : *The
Psychology of Open Teaching and Learning* : Little
Brown, Boston.

Rogers, C.R. 1983 *Freedom to Learn for the Eighties* :
Merrill, Columbus, Ohio.

Rogers, C.R. 1985 Towards a More Human Science of the
Person : *Journal of Humanistic Psychology* : 25 : 7 -
24.

Rolfe, G. 1990 The Role of Clinical Supervision in the
Education of Student Psychiatric Nurses : a
Theoretical Approach : *Nurse Education Today* : 10 :
193 - 197.

Roszak, T. 1969 *The Making of a Counter Culture :
Reflections on the Technocratic Society and its
Youthful Opposition* : Doubleday : New York.

Rowan, J. 1988 *Ordinary Ecstasy : Humanistic Psychology in
Action* : 2nd Edition : Routledge, London.

Rowan, J. 1989 The Self : One or Many? *The Psychologist : Bulletin of the British Psychological Society* : : 7 : 279 - 281.

Rowan, J. and Dryden, W. 1989 *Innovative Therapy in Britain* : Open University Press, Milton Keynes.

Rowntree, D. 1988 *Assessing Students : How Shall We Know Them?* : 2nd Edition : Harper and Row, London.

Ryle, G. 1949 *The Concept of Mind* : Peregrine, Harmondsworth.

Salvage, J. 1985 *The Politics of Nursing* : Heinemann, London.

Sankar, S. 1987 Teaching Psychiatric Nursing : Curriculum Development for the 1982 Syllabus. In B.D. Davis (ed) *Nursing Education : Research and Developments* : Croom Helm, London.

Sartre, J-P, 1955 *Being and Nothingness* : Philosophical Library : New York.

Schafer, B.P. and Morgan, M.K. 1980 An Experiential Learning Laboratory : A New Dimension in Teaching Mental Health Skills : *Issues in Mental Health Nursing* : 2 : 3 : 47 - 57.

Schon, D.A. 1983 *The Reflective Practitioner : How Professionals Think in Action* : Temple Smith, London.

Schutz, W.C. 1967 *Joy* : Grove Press, New York.

Schutz, W.C. 1971 *Here Comes Everybody* : Harper and Row, New York.

Schutz, W.C. 1973 *Elements of Encounter* : Irvington Publishers, New York.

Scott, C. 1961 Research on Mail Surveys : *Journal of the Royal Statistical Society* : XXIV : Series A : 143 - 195.

Shaffer, J.B.P. 1978 *Humanistic Psychology* : Prentice Hall, Englewood Cliffs, New Jersey.

Shapiro, S.B. 1985 An Empirical Analysis of Operating Values in Humanistic Psychology : *Journal of Humanistic Psychology* : 25 : 1 : 94 - 108.

Sigel, J. and Scipio-Skinner, K.V. 1983 Psychodrama : an experiential model for nursing students : *Group Psychotherapy, Psychodrama and Sociometry* : 36 : 97 - 101.

Simon, S, Howe,E. and Kirschenbaum, H. 1978 *Values Clarification* : 2nd Edition : A & W Visual Library, New York.

Smith, P.B. 1980 *Group Processes and Personal Change* : Harper and Row, London.

Spradley J.A. 1979 *Participant Observation* : Holt, Rinehart and Winston, New York

Steinaker, N.W. and Bell, M.R. 1979 *The Experiential Taxonomy : a new approach to teaching and learning* : Academic Press, New York.

Stevens, J.O. 1971 *Awareness : Exploring, Experimenting, Exploring* : Real People Press, Moab, Utah.

Stern, P.N. 1985 Using Grounded Theory Method in Nursing Research. In M.M. Leninger (ed) *Qualitative Research Methods in Nursing* : Grune and Stratton, New York

Strauss, A.L. 1986 *Qualitative Data Analysis for Social Scientists* : Cambridge University Press, Cambridge.

Tomlinson. A. 1985 The Use of Experiential Methods in Teaching Interpersonal Skills to Nurses. In C.M. Kagan (ed) *Interpersonal Skills in Nursing : Research and Applications* : Croom Helm, London.

Treece, E.W. and Treece, J.W. 1977 *Elements of Research in Nursing* : C.V. Mosby, New York.

Trudgill, P. 1983 *Sociolinguistics : An Introduction to Language and Society* : Penguin, Harmondsworth.

Tschudin, V. 1986 *Ethics in Nursing : The Caring Relationship* : Heinemann, London.

Tschudin, V. 1986 *Counselling Skills for Nurses* : 2nd Edition : Balliere Tindall, London.

Turabian, K.L. 1987 *A Manual for Writers of Term Papers, Theses and Dissertations* : University of Chicago Press, Chicago.

Turk, C. and Kirkman, J. 1989 *Effective Writing : Improving Scientific, Technical and Business Communication* : 2nd Edition : E. and F.N. Spon, London.

Van Maanen, J. 1983 *Qualitative Methodology* : Sage, Beverly Hills, California.

Van Ments, M. 1983 *The Effective Use of Role-Play* : Kogan Page, London.

Vaughan, B. and Pillmoor, M. 1989 *Managing Nursing Work* : Scutari Press, London.

Walker, D. 1985 Writing and Reflection. In D. Boud, R. Keogh and D. Walker. *Reflection : Turning Experience into Learning* : Kogan Page, London.

Wallis, R. 1984 *The Elementary Forms of the New Religious Life* : Routledge and Kegan Paul, London.

Walsh, K.K., VandenBosch, T.M. and Boehm, S. 1989 Modelling and Role Modeling : Integrating Nursing Theory and Practice : *Journal of Advanced Nursing* : 14 : 755 - 761.

Watkins, R. and Addison, J. (1990) All the World's a Stage : *Nursing Times* : 86 : 21 : 47 - 48.

Webb, E.J.D.T., Cambell, R.D., Schwartz, R.D. and Sechrest, L. 1966 *Unobtrusive Measures* : Rand McNally, Chicago.

Weill, S.W. and McGill, I. (eds) 1989 *Making Sense of Experiential Learning : Diversity in Theory and Practice* : Open University Press, Milton Keynes.

Weiss, A.R. and Kempler, B. 1986 The Role of Intent in Psychological Research : *Journal of Humanistic Psychology* : 26 : 1 : 117 - 125.

Whitaker, D.S. 1987 *Using Groups to Help People* : Tavistock/Routledge, London.

Whitehead, A.N. 1922 *The Aims of Education* : Benn, London.

Wibley, S. 1983 The Use of Role Play : *Nursing Mirror* : June 22nd : 54 - 55.

Wilber, K. 1981 *Up from Eden : A Transpersonal View of Human Evolution* : Routledge and Kegan Paul, London.

Williams, B. 1973 *The Problems of Self* : OUP, Oxford.

Wilson, C. 1956 *The Outsider* : Gollanzc, London

Wittgenstein, L. 1961 (1922) *Tractatus Logico-Philosophicus* : Routledge and Kegan Paul, London.

Woolfe, R., Dryden, W. and Charles-Edwards, D. 1989 The Nature and Range of Counselling Practice. In W. Dryden, D. Charles-Edwards and R. Woolfe (eds) : *Handbook of Counselling in Britain* : Routledge, London.

Worf, B.J. 1956 *Language, Thought and Reality : Selected Writings* : Technology Press of Massachusetts Institute of Technology : Cambridge, Mass.

Wright Mills, C. 1959 *The Sociological Imagination* : Oxford University Press, Oxford.

Wright, S. 1990 *My Patient-My Nurse* : Scutari, London.
Yalom, I.D. 1977 Existential Psychotherapy. In O.L. McCabe
(ed) *Changing Human Behaviour* : Grune and Stratton,
New York.
Youngman, M.B. 1978 *Designing and Analysing Questionnaires*
: Nottingham University School of Education,
Nottingham.

Bibliography

Other Publications By Philip Burnard

Books

Burnard, P. 1985 **Learning Human Skills : a Guide for Nurses**
: Heinemann, London.
Burnard, P. 1986 **Self-Awareness for Nurses : an Experiential
Guide** : Aspen, Rockville, Maryland.
Burnard, P. and Chapman, C. 1988 **Professional and Ethical
Issues in Nursing : the Code of Professional Conduct :**
Wiley, Chichester.
Burnard, P. 1989 **Counselling Skills for Health Professionals :**
Chapman and Hall, London.
Burnard, P. 1989 **Teaching Interpersonal Skills : a Handbook
of Experiential Learning for Health Professionals :**
Chapman and Hall, London.
Burnard, P. and Chapman, C. 1990 **Nurse Education : The
Way Forward** : Scutari, London.
Burnard, P. and Morrison, P. 1990 **Nursing Research in
Action : Developing Basic Skills** : Macmillan, London.
Burnard, P. 1990 **Learning Human Skills : An Experiential
Guide for Nurses** : 2nd Edition : Heinemann, London.

Burnard, P. Coping With Stress in the Health Professions : a
Practical Guide : Chapman and Hall, London.

Chapters in Books

Burnard, P. 1987 Facing Change Through Self-Awareness. In
ENB Learning Package : **Managing Change in Nurse
Education** : English National Board for Nursing, Mid-
wifery and Health Visiting, London.
Burnard, P. 1990 Six chapters. In E.M. Horne (ed) : **Effective
Communication** : Austen Cornish, London.
Burnard, P. 1990 Two chapters. In E.M. Horne (ed) : **The
Staff Nurse's Survival Guide** : Austen Cornish, London.
Burnard, P. 1990 Two chapters. In E.M. Horne (ed) : **The
Ward Sister's Survival Guide** : Austen Cornish, London.
Burnard, P. 1990 Meaningful Dialogue. In R. L. Ismeurt, F.N.
Arnold and Carson, V.B. 1990 **Readings in Concepts
Fundamental to Nursing** : Springhouse, Pennsylvania.

Papers and Articles

Burnard, P. 1983 Through Experience and From Experience :
Nursing Mirror : 156 : 9 : 29 - 33.
Burnard, P. 1984 The Human Potential Movement : a Per-
sonal Perspective : **Self and Society : The European
Journal of Humanistic Psychology** : xii : 2 : 28 - 34.
Burnard, P. 1984 Developing Self-Awareness : **Nursing Mirror**
: 158 : 21 : 30 -31.
Burnard, P. 1984 The Way Forward : **Senior Nurse** : 1 : 12 :
14 - 18.
Burnard, P. 1984 Counselling the Counsellors : **Senior Nurse** :
1 : 13 : 15 - 19.
Burnard, P. 1984 Training to Be Aware : **Senior Nurse** : 1 : 23
: 25 - 27.
Burnard, P. 1984 A Setback for Psychiatric Nurse Training? :
Nursing times : 80 : 49 : 53 - 54.
Burnard, P. 1984 Paradigms for Progress : **Senior Nurse** : 1 :
38 : 24 - 26.
Bailey, C., Burnard, P. and Smith, R. 1985 Breaking the Ice :
Nursing Mirror : 160 : 1 : 26 - 28.

Burnard, P. 1985 Future Imperfect? : **Senior Nurse** : 2 : 1 : 8 -
     11.
Burnard, P. 1985 Stop, Look and Listen. : **Senior Nurse** : 2 : 9
     : 21 - 22.
Burnard, P. 1985 Teacher as Facilitator : **Senior Nurse** : 2 : 9
     : 34 - 37.
Burnard, P. 1985 Listening to People : **Nursing Mirror** : 16 :18
     : 28 - 29.
Burnard, P. 1985 Learning to Communicate : **Nursing Mirror** :
     16: 19 : 30 - 31.
Burnard, P. 1985 How to Reduce Stress : **Nursing Mirror** : 16 :
     19 : 47 - 48.
Burnard, P. 1986 Encountering Adults : **Senior Nurse** : 4 : 4 : 30
     - 31.
Burnard, P. 1986 Learning About Groups : **Nurse Education Today**   :
     6 : 116 - 120.
Burnard, P. 1986 Picking Up the Pieces : **Nursing Times** : 82 :
     17 : 37 -39.
Burnard, P. 1986 Hazard, Tutor at Work : **Senior Nurse** : 5 : 5 -
     6.
Burnard, P. 1987 Towards an Epistemological Basis for
     Experiential Learning : **Journal of Advanced Nursing** : 12
     : 189 - 193.
Burnard, P. 1987 Spiritual Distress and the Nursing Response :
     Theoretical Considerations and Counselling Skills :
     Journal of Advanced Nursing : 12 : 377 - 382.
Burnard, P. 1987 Meditation : Uses and Methods in Psychiatric
     Nurse Education : **Nurse Education Today** : 7 : 4 : 191 -
     197.
Burnard, P. 1987 Coping With Emotion in Intensive Care
     Nursing : **Intensive Care Nursing** : 3 : 4 : 157 - 159.
Burnard, P. 1987 Playing the Game : **Nursing Times** : 13 : 61 -
     62.
Burnard, P. 1987 Meaningful Dialogue : **Nursing Times** : 83 : 20
     : 43 - 45.
Burnard, P. 1987 Self and Peer Assessment : **Senior Nurse**: 6 :
     5 : 16 - 17.
Burnard, P. 1987 Counselling : Basic Principles in Nursing : **The
     Professional Nurse** : 2 : 9 : 278 - 280.
Burnard, P. 1987 The Right Direction : **Senior Nurse** : 7 : 1 :
     30-32.

Burnard, P. 1987 The Health Visitor as Counsellor : a Framework for Interpersonal SKills : **Health Visitor** : 60 : 8 : 269.

Burnard, P. 1987 Interpersonal Skills : Sharing a Viewpoint : **Senior Nurse** : 7 : 3 : 38 - 39.

Burnard, P. and Morrison, P. 1987 Nurses' Perceptions of Their Interpersonal Skills : **Nursing Times** : 83 : 42 : 59.

Burnard, P. 1986 Integrated Self-Awareness Training : a holistic model : **Nurse Education Today** : 6 : 219 - 222.

Burnard, P. 1986 Psychiatric Nurse Education : a Question of Balance? : **Nurse Education Today** : 6 : 215 - 218.

Burnard, P. 1987 Developing Skills as a Group Facilitator : **The Professional Nurse** : 3 : 1 : 19 - 21.

Burnard, P. 1987 Nurse Education in the USA : **Senior Nurse** : 7 . 5 . 27 38.

Burnard, P. 1987 Teaching the Teachers : **Nursing Times** : 83 : 49 : 63 -65.

Burnard, P. 1987 Counselling Skills : **Journal of District Nursing** : 6 : 7 : 12 - 14.

Burnard, P. 1987 Nurse Educators and Experiential Learning : **Nursing Times** : 84 : 2 : 56.

Burnard, P. 1987 Learning to Listen : **Journal of District Nursing** : 6 : 9 : 26 - 28.

Burnard, P. 1988 The Journal as an Assessment and Evaluation Tool in Nurse Education : **Nurse Education Today** : 8 : 105 - 107.

Burnard, P. 1988 Self Evaluation Methods in Nurse Education : **Nurse Education Today** : 8 : 229 - 233.

Burnard, P. 1988 Self-Awareness and Intensive Care Nursing : **Intensive Care Nursing** : 4 : 67 - 70.

Burnard, P. 1988 Experiential Learning : Some Theoretical Considerations : **International Journal of Lifelong Education** : 7 : 2 : 127 - 133.

Burnard, P. and Morrison, P. 1988 Nurses' Perceptions of Their Interpersonal Skills : a Descriptive Study Using Six Category Intervention Analysis : **Nurse Education Today** : 8 : 266 - 272.

Burnard, P. 1988 'Brainstorming' : A Practical Learning Activity in Nurse Education : **Nurse Education Today** : 8 : 354 - 358.

Burnard, P. 1988 Communicating on the Telephone : **Senior Nurse** : 8 : 13 : 14 - 18.

Burnard, P. 1988 Self-Awareness : **Journal of District Nursing** : 6 : 10 : 27 - 29.

Burnard, P. 1988 Emotional Release : **Journal of District Nursing** : 6 : 11 : 26 - 28.

Burnard, P. 1988 Developing Counselling SKills in Health Visitors : an Experiential Approach : **Health Visitor** : 61 : 5 : 20 - 23.

Burnard, P. 1988 Building on Experience : **Senior Nurse** : 8 : 5 : 18 - 20.

Burnard, P. 1988 Four Dimensions in Counselling : **Nursing Times** : 84 : 20 : 37 - 39.

Burnard, P. 1988 No Need to Hide : **Nursing Times** : 84 : 24 : 36 - 38.

Morrison, P. and Burnard, P. 1988 Clarifying Nurses' Inter-personal Skills : **Nursing Times** : 84 : 30 : 49.

Burnard, P. 1988 Searching for Meaning : **Nursing Times** : 84 : 37 : 34 - 36.

Burnard, P. 1988 AIDS and Sexuality : **Journal of District Nursing** : 7 : 2 : 7 - 8.

Burnard, P. 1988 Empathy : The Key to Understanding : **The Professional Nurse** : 3 : 10 : 388 - 392.

Burnard, P. 1988 Self-Directed Learning : **Journal of District Nursing** : 7 ;1; 7 - 8.

Burnard, P. 1988 Coping With Other People's Emotions : **The Professional Nurse** : 4 : 1 : 11- 14.

Burnard, P. 1988 Preventing Burnout : **Journal of District Nursing** : 7 : 5 : 9 - 10.

Burnard, P. 1988 Mentors : a Supporting Act : **Nursing Times** : 84 : 46 : 27 - 28.

Burnard, P. 1988 Discussing Spiritual Issues With Clients : **Health Visitor** : 61 : 12 : 371 - 372.

Burnard, P. 1988 The Spiritual Needs of Atheists and Agnostics : **The Professional Nurse** : 4 : 3 : 130 - 132.

Burnard, P. 1988 Stress and Relaxation in Health Visiting : **Health Visitor** : 61 : 12 : 272.

Burnard, P. 1988 The Heart of the Counselling Relationship : **Senior Nurse** : 8 : 12 : 17 - 18.

Burnard, P. 1988 Equality and Meaning : Issues in the Interpersonal Relationship : **Community Psychiatric
Nursing Journal** : 8 : 6 : 17 - 21.

Burnard, P. 1989 Exploring Nurse Educators' Views of
Experiential Learning : a Pilot Study : **Nurse Education Today** : 9 : 1 : 39 -45.

Burnard, P. 1989 Developing Critical Ability in Nurse Education : **Nurse Education Today** : 9 : 271 - 275.

Burnard, P. 1989 Experiential Learning and Andragogy -
Negotiated Learning in Nurse Education : a Critical
Appraisal : **Nurse Education Today** : 9 : 5 : 300 - 306.

Morrison, P. and Burnard, P. 1989 Students' and Trained
Nurses' Perceptions of Their Own Interpersonal Skills :
a report and comparison : **Journal of Advanced
Nursing** : 14 : 321 - 329.

Burnard, P. 1989 Pitventiunum us A Theoretical Basis for
Counselling in Psychiatric Nursing : **Archives of
Psychiatric Nursing** : III : 3 : 142 - 147.

Burnard, P. and Morrison, P. 1989 What is an Interpersonally
Skilled Person? : A Repertory Grid Account of
Professional Nurses' Views : **Nurse Education Today** :
9 : 6 : 384 - 391.

Burnard, P. 1989 Psychiatric Nursing Students' Perceptions
of Experiential Learning : **Nursing Times** : 85 : 1 : 52.

Burnard, P. 1989 The Role of Mentor : **Journal of District
Nursing** : 8 : 3 : 8 - 10.

Burnard, P. 1989 Exploring Sexuality : **Journal of District
Nursing** : 8 : 4 : 9 - 11.

Burnard, P. 1989 Counselling in Surgical Nursing : **Surgical
Nurse** : 2 : 5 : 12 - 14.

Burnard, P. and Morrison, P. 1989 Client-Centred Approach :
Nursing Times : 85 : 15 : 60 - 61.

Burnard, P. and Morrison, P. 1989 Counselling Attitudes in
Community Psychiatric Nurses : **Community
Psychiatric Nursing Journal** : 9 : 5 : 26 - 29.

Burnard, P. 1989 The Nurse as Non-Conformist : **Nursing
Standard** : 4 : 1 : 32 - 35.

Burnard, P. 1989 Exploring Nurses' Attitudes to AIDS : **The
Professional Nurse** : 5 : 2 : 84 - 90.

Burnard, P. 1989 Learning From the Learners : **Nursing Standard** : 4 : 6 : 26 - 27.

Burnard, P. 1989 The 'Sixth Sense' : **Nursing Times** : 85 : 50 : 52 - 53.

Burnard, P. 1990 Counselling the Boss : **Nursing Times** : 86 : 1 : 58 - 59.

Burnard, P. 1990 Counselling in Crises : **Journal of District Nursing** : 8 : 7 : 15 - 16.

Burnard, P. 1990 Learning to Care for the Spirit : **Nursing Standard** : 4 : 18 : 38 - 39.

Burnard, P. 1990 Thoughts About Theories : **Nursing Standard** : 4 : 21 : 47.

Burnard, P. 1990 Staying in Balance : Humanistic Psychology and Psychiatric Nursing : **Community Psychiatric Nursing Journal** : 10 : 1 : 16 -19.

Burnard, P. 1990 Recording Counselling in Nursing : **Senior Nurse** : 10 : 3 : 26 - 27.

Morrison, P. and Burnard, P. 1990 Interpersonal Skills : A Smallest Space Analysis : **Nursing Times** : 86 : 14 : 55.

Burnard, P. 1990 Critical Awareness in Nurse Education : **Nursing Standard** : 4 : 30 : 32 - 34.

Burnard, P. 1990 Problems With M.E. : **Journal of District Nursing** : 8 : 12 : 22 - 23.

Burnard, P. 1990 Ambivalence in Humanistic Psycholgy : **Self and Society : The European Journal of Humanistic Psychology** : XVIII : 3 : 40 - 41.

Burnard, P. 1990 Is Anyone Here a Mentor? : **Nursing Standard** : 4 : 37 : 46.

Burnard, P. 1990 The Supervisory Role : **Journal of District Nursing** : July : 26 - 27.

Burnard, P. 1990 The Orton Experience : **Nursing Times** : 86 : 32 : 56 - 57.

Burnard, P. and Morrison, P. 1990 Psychological Aspects of Self-Esteem : **Surgical Nurse** : 3 : 4 : 4 - 6.

Burnard, P. 1990 Group Discussion : **Nursing Times** : 12 : 86 : 36 - 37.

Burnard, P. 1990 Using Experiential Teaching Methods : **Nursing Times** : 86 : 41 : 53.

Burnard, P. 1990 **So You Think You Need a Computer ?** : The Professional Nurse : 6 : 2 : 119 - 120.

Burnard, P. and Morrison, P. 1990 Counselling Attitudes in Health Visiting Students : **Health Visitor** : 63 : 11 : 389 - 390.

Burnard, P. 1990 The Student Experience : Adult Learning
and Mentorship Revisited : **Nurse Education Today** : 10
: 5 : 349 - 353.

Burnard, P. 1990 Stating the Case : **Counselling : The Journal
of the British Association for Counselling** : 1 : 4 :
114 - 116.

Burnard,P. 1990 Exploring Meaninglessness : **Journal of
District Nursing** : 9 : 6 : 10 - 13.

Burnard, P. 1990 The Cult of the Personality : **Nursing
Standard** : 5 : 14 : 46 - 47.

Burnard, P. 1991 Computing : An Aid to Studying Nursing :
Nursing Standard : 5 : 17 : 36 - 38.

Burnard, P. 1991 Exploring Personal Values : **Journal of
District Nursing** : 9 : 7 : 7 - 8.

Burnard, P. and Morrison, P. 1991 Nurses' Interpersonal Skills
: a Study of Nurses' Perceptions : **Nurse Education
Today** : 11 : 1 : 24 - 29.

Burnard, P. 1991 Peer Support Groups : **Journal of District
Nursing** : 9 : 8 : 19 - 20.

Burnard, P. 1991 Perceptions of Experiential Learning :
Nursing Times : 87 : 8 : 47.

Burnard, P. 1991 Interpersonal Skills Training : **Journal of
District Nursing** : 9 : 10 : 17 - 20.

Burnard, P. 1991 Improving Through Reflection : **Journal of
District Nursing** : 9 : 11 : 10 - 12.

Burnard, P. and Morrison, P. 1991 Client-Centred Counselling
: A Study of Nurses' Attitudes : **Nurse Education
Today** : 11 : 104 - 109.

Burnard, P. 1991 Using Video as a Reflective Tool in
Interpersonal Skills Training : **Nurse Education Today** :
11 : 143 - 146.

Index